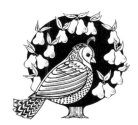

Immunology
of the Soul
The Paradigm
for the Future

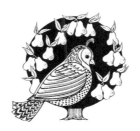

Immunology
of the Soul
The Paradigm
for the Future

Ursula M. Anderson, M.D.

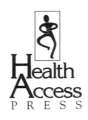

Health
Access
PRESS

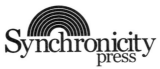

Synchronicity
press

Sanford • Florida

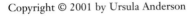

Published by InSync Communications LLC, Health Access Press, and Synchronicity Press
2445 River Tree Circle
Sanford, FL 32771
http://www.insynchronicity.com

This book was set in Adobe Janson Text
Cover Design and Composition by Jonathan Pennell

Library of Congress Catalog Number: 00-103409
        Anderson. Ursula M.,
Immunology of the Soul
        ISBN: 1-929902-02-6

First Health Access Press and Synchronicity Press Edition
10 9 8 7 6 5 4 3 2 1
Printed in the United States of America

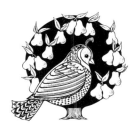

Dedication

To the Memories that arrived with me
on Planet Earth.

To memories that the living of my life
rendered to me.

To those souls whose energies collided
with mine to make my journey bumpy,
and to those who souls encountering mine made the road
smooth.

But above all
to the children who
in the smooth and bumpy times
taught me that Love and Hope,
and belief in their existence,
is a ceaseless call and a
neverending unfolding of the
Consciousness of Life Divine.

I give my loving gratitude.

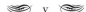

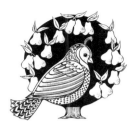

Publisher's Comments

J UST AS THIS BOOK WAS GOING TO PRESS the media came alive with stories about the cracking of the Genome. *Newsweek*, *Time*, *ABC* and *NBC*, *CBS*, *CNN*, and the *BBC*, the Internet, collegiate newspapers — they all carried major stories on the significance of the mapping of the 3.1 billion chemical "letters" that make up human DNA. Some equated this event to the first moon landing (which interestingly enough took place nearly thirty-one years to the day). Others looked upon this cosmic, yet earthly event as something as historically critical as the invention of the printing press or discovery of the wheel.

What Dr. Ursula Anderson has accomplished in ***Immunology of the Soul: The Paradigm for the Future***, is something quite challenging to the mindset that many of us have been programmed to establish for ourselves. Likewise, her challenges come wrapped up in a most extraordinary format. In light of the Human Genome Project, Dr. Anderson's book becomes ever more extraordinary. Between its covers is woven a journey through the yet to be explored territories of what turns the genome "on," what actually drives it, and what turns it "against" its intended healthy functioning in the form of diseases and dysfunctions of the body, mind and soul.

The author's persistent invitation for the reader to look to *energy* and its constant and cosmic dance with *memory* and *consciousness* as the ultimate secret in the glory and aberration of whom we truly are (and thus becomes the power that maintains and/or alters the human genome), reminded me of the holiday song that recounts the giving of various gifts over the twelve days of Christmas. You may recall that it starts with a partridge in a pear tree and ends each portion of the round with the same phrase. The strong symbolic image and virtual importance of this partridge is the glue that brings all the other gifts together and serves as the underlying unity in the song. The metaphor is that throughout history and in all avenues of inquiry pursued by scientific and spiritual seekers — and despite the many gifts of insight and knowledge that we've obtained — the constant that threads throughout and holds things together is that so much still begs for answers: that being the very nature and dynamics of life and the infinity of its expression.

Immunology of the Soul should serve as a pure stimulant to the appetite for such answers. And in doing so, it invites the reader to a banquet of what we *may* become if we address the redressing of human disease and dysfunction of our bodies, minds and souls — within the context of their sacredness, as the author suggests. Eric Lander, head of the Whitehead-M.I.T. Center for Genome Research, quoted in *Newsweek*, remarked that "who finishes first is not as important as what happens next." In an interview with *TIME*, he was quoted as saying that "the important issues are as much social and philosophical as they are scientific." He went on to discuss our mutual human roots: Our species has only a modest amount of genetic variation — the DNA of any two humans is 99.9% identical. I'm not such a Pollyanna as to think that merely knowing this will put an end to ethnic strife, but I hope it will influence our thinking. The more we understand the human genetic tapestry, the more we see that our similarities outweigh our differences."

It is possible that this may serve to explain the graphic used in this book — the persistence of a partridge in a pear tree!

— **Dennis N. McClellan**
Publisher

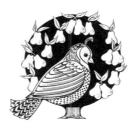

Contents

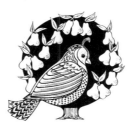

Acknowledgements

Immunology of the Soul:
The Paradigm for the Future

THIS BOOK IS THE THIRD VOLUME of a trilogy I have written over the last three years, The Psalms of Children: Their Songs and Laments being the first and Connections, the second. Each emerged from the same lineage of concern for the escalation of violence throughout the world and, in particular, among the young. Each in its own way describes the pivotal role that memory, both personal and trans-generational, has played in the evolution of human consciousness and how both play out in human feelings and behavior. Overall, they issue an invitation to re-think whom we are and how we came to be whom we are. Immunology of the Soul goes further by exposing the beliefs and attitudes that have blighted the divine within our human nature. In so doing, it gives promise to what we may become if we put our hands to the plough of tending the soil of the communal human soul. Such knowledge comes from the interplay of many energies — intuition, observation, people, places, books, art, music, and customs, to mention but a few. Throughout my journey, they have been my constant companions and all, in one way or another, have been my teachers. So, I acknowledge and give thanks for their tutelage of the ways of light and dark. They were, in fact, gifts of the One, Eternal, and Holy Spirit who travels with us all and who is, therefore, above all the source of my knowledge and the recipient of my gratitude.

I have again been blessed with the loving assistance of James Doyle, M.Div. who transformed my handwritten text into a readable and computer-friendly text. Thank you, James, and may the angels surprise you with many blessings.

Several of my friends and colleagues took time from their busy lives to read the manuscript and render previews; they and others have given formidable support for its messages. In this regard, special thanks flow to Dr. Billy Andrews, Dr. Richard Cox, Dr, Edith Fiore, Dr. Robert Jonas, Professor Asphodel Long, Dr. John Allen Loftus, Mrs. Eleanor May-Brenneker, Dr. Christine Page and Dr. Ovey Mohammed. To those others not specifically mentioned, as well as to Mr. Chris Kwiat and Ms. Roslyne Mandeville for their logistical support, my sincere thanks. Special gratitude goes to Dr. Wayne Teasdale of the World Parliament of Religions for his sensitive foreword, which fastens so well to the messages and intent of this book.

To all, within all, and through all, may the oneness of the God of All be praised and made manifest!

Ursula M. Anderson

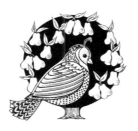

Foreword

MOTHER TERESA WAS ONCE ASKED by a journalist why she does what she does. That is, why she loves the unlovable by fishing babies out of gutters and off street corners, operates homes and orphanages for children, and cares for the dying poor. The saint responded: "It is because I realized I had a Hitler inside me." Mother Teresa's love immunized her against the self-enclosed world of the egotist and the thick, uncaring insensitivity of that world, which like a fatal disease, destroys any hope of a life of heroic virtue. All of us at one time or another — if we are honest — have to admit that we also have this same potential for evil and selfishness from which we can only be rescued by grace and a good will.

Ursula Anderson, drawing on all her wisdom as a doctor of the soul, and using the metaphors of medicine and spirituality, lays bare the threats to the soul and to human identity to achieve its potential for wholeness, integrity, depth, and spiritual maturity. Her years as a pediatrician and a psychiatrist, coupled with wisdom gained in her own inner life on the spiritual journey, have uniquely positioned her intellectually, intuitively, culturally, and morally to attain and develop those rich insights present in this volume. She takes the care of the soul far beyond Thomas Moore's popular and much appreciated contribution, exposing the root causes of why the soul, or human identity, is under pressure and attack from so many negative forces in our time, and really in all ages. For if the soul, the gem of human awareness, is to be immunized, or protected from these lethal psychological influences that translate themselves into dangerous actions in society, then we must know the nature and causes of these diseases. At the same time, we must have genuine knowledge of the soul's nature — the incomparable greatness of which the human person is capable when freed from harmful social and psychological pathogens.

All of the great founders of humankind's religious traditions were actually physicians of the soul, in their own way engaging in the difficult and subtle science/art of soul-craft, of depth spiritual direction, stretching the human to activate and realize its potential for divinity. That potential is only actualized and fully realized in a life when the person, the *soul*, surrenders to holiness, or the perfection of compassion, kindness, mercy, sensitivity, and love. It is not enough to merely be immunized, as Ursula Anderson makes clear, but this protection is only a first step, a *sine qua non*, for the real growth and health of the soul to occur. In a very real sense, we see the truly healthy soul, the genuinely integrated and aware person, in the saint, the moral hero of all our spiritual schools.

Our need for healing is so obvious, our nature so profound, and the threats to it so terrifying, that a contribution of the quality of Dr. Anderson's is greatly needed in our time. Her understanding of human nature, her sensitive and holistic insights into children, and her intuitions of direction for the future of humanity individually and collectively make this book particularly timely. This is a work motivated by dedication and love. It reminds me of something the Dalai Lama once said to an aggressive reporter who had asked him what his religion was all about. He wanted to know what made this Buddhist icon tick. His Holiness looked at the reporter with love and humor and eloquently remarked, "It's really quite simple. My religion is kindness. My religion is kindness." A Christian might say, "My religion is love. My religion is love." Ursula Anderson, in her own way, adds to this insight and this task for humankind — the transformation of souls into love.

Brother Wayne Teasdale, Ph.D.,
World Parliament of Religions, Chicago

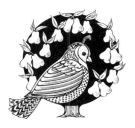

Prologue

W E LIVE IN A WORLD wherein single words, and the concepts they symbolize, have become so entrenched in popular usage that we may have put ourselves at risk of diminishing the substance of their essential meaning. Immunology and soul are two such words. Soul has recently received a lot of attention and examination and, heaven knows, so has immunology. Rendered in copious garbs of how to protect and enhance the immune system, these nobly intentioned gems of bookly wisdom instruct the plebs on how to delay entrance into heaven's paradise, if not also how to minimize the hells of living and personal experience before they get there. Yet, if we juxtapose the one with the other, we discover they share an essential interdependence, one that hitherto through all the hype has lain fallow. Let me explain.

To be immunized means to be protected against attack on self and self-identity by that which would otherwise cripple, disable, or destroy us.

Immunology is the science and study of the means whereby we are or can be defended against that which being non-self seeks to intrude on self and/or self-identity and injure or take them away in part or in whole. So far, immunology has placed emphasis on understanding the mechanisms underlying natural immunity to physical disease and discovering and developing the means to protect against their ravages. This latter has been and continues to be achieved predominantly through vaccines which have proven spectacularly successful and whose *modus operandi* basically depends on altering the memories of engagement between the attacker and the attackee.

But, we are more than our bodies. We are trinities of body, mind, and soul and the memories that reside within the human soul are the matrix from which human behavior ensues. Presently, the killing fields of humankind derive from disorders of human behavior whose causes reside in the dis-eases and dys-functions of the soul.

All over the world, violence and wars are taking their toll in homes, families, and neighborhoods, as are enmities between religious and ethnic groups and nations. Because we are one creation and carry within us a shared consciousness, the fallout from massive displacement, starvation and epidemics heaped onto countless personal tragedies reaches all sectors of society around the globe. Likewise, the greed that mindlessly exploits the treasures of the earth for the enrichment of a few impoverishes all of us and threatens not only outer ecological balance but also the inner ecology of the communal human soul.

If physical diseases can be ameliorated, prevented, and even eliminated by immunization procedures, which in essence change the nature and texture of the soil in their battlegrounds and, thus, the memories and energies of their engagement, then surely this can also be accomplished for diseases of the soul. Applying the principles of immunology to this great task requires first an understanding of the texture of the soil wherein these battles are fought and the nature of the assailants that engage its memories and energies. Then, and only then, will we be able to embark on the odyssey whose ports of call are the soils of the belief systems that caused the battles and the havens wherein the wounds of their casualties may be healed. These are the messages of the

Immunology of the Soul

and

The Hope of New Paradigms for the Future

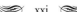

I

The Soil of Soul

I T IS NO SECRET THAT VIOLENCE is ripping apart the fabric of society all over the world. So terrible is its devastation that the United Nations has been called upon to declare the years 2000 through 2010 the decade for the culture of non-violence. This appeal has been made by the Nobel Peace Laureates to all member states, and they further requested that the year 2000 be declared a year for education in peace and non-violence. In a recorded message to those assembled at the press conference where this initiative was announced, Aung San Suis Kyi, winner of the 1991 Nobel Peace Prize, stated that one of the best possible contributions toward peace and security in the world would be to help children build healthy, joyful lives. Violence against children, she said, constituted violence against the best in ourselves.

The truth of what this great lady and human rights activist says is self-evident, for when children are spared their lives and become adults, they bring to their adult behavior the memories and consciousness of their childhood experiences. And, yet, this fundamental knowledge about human behavior appears to be little known and even less appreciated in terms of what a commitment to it could achieve for humankind.

Evidence of this resides in the rumors originating in the adult world that children are to blame for violence, and, there is a ground-swell of indignation against this generation of so-called predators who kill and maim and are violent beyond what is known or thought to be known about previous generations. How do these conflicting beliefs arise? Where does it all come from? How did violence itself get started on its journey of destruction?

Let me start to tease it apart by inviting you to share a wintry day in my office in the year 1995. Despite the inclement weather, it had been a very busy morning and the schedule planned for the afternoon promised a repeat of the morning. So, instead of taking a break for lunch, I started compiling my evaluations and recommendations for the children I had so far seen that day.

Preparing these reports is a task that invariably calls forth a medley of concerns and compassion. The majority of children referred to me have been born into family and home situations that would take the wisdom of a Solomon to handle, let alone resolve; many have learning as well as emotional, and behavioral difficulties and all too frequently they are saddled with all of these burdens. Additionally, if not invariably, many have been physically, verbally, emotionally and/or sexually abused, and all have endured injury to their souls wherein reside feelings, as well as the seed — if not also the flower — of our own unique sense of identity. I usually begin our encounters by asking the children to tell me what they believe to be the cause of their problems and what measures they think should be taken to lessen or resolve them. This helps not only to establish trust, but renders significant insights into the dynamics of their lives. Most importantly, it conveys a willingness to listen and for them to be heard, of itself therapeutic in as much as without exception they believe and feel, and not without cause, that no one listens to them, and that they have little say or control over their lives.

Predictably, they tell me they want to be free to be their own person, free of all strictures regardless the means that would be necessary to remove them and, since we live in a society where money is equated with power and control, money, and lots of it, features prominently in their wish lists. Yet, however loaded with material wants and assets these lists become, without exception, the common denominator they wish for most is to be and to feel connected to their birth-families, from whom they are frequently permanently or temporarily disconnected, and to be and to feel loved and valued just for being whom they are as their own person. All too often when they rebel against the circumstances that, through no fault of their own, denies this to them, their rebellious behavior is perceived by those who exercise control over them as the "major" or "central" problem requiring correction. Thus, they become victimized twice. Perceiving the child as the problem rather than as a sentient individual reacting, often very appropriately to the problems of their parents, families or their surrogates, makes of the child's dearest aspirations and wishes the extreme end of what is not possible. Sadly, this is verified by the repetitive contacts so many have with a variety of agencies and professionals, all neatly indexed and documented, though with little reference to wholesome outcome in the voluminous reports that accompany them to my office. Juxtaposing the many words why's, wherefore's, and conjectures contained therein, with my own findings, diagnoses, and recommendations demands more than a rational rearrangement of the whole though of course this often helps.

In the process, I find myself searching in a meditative way for remedies to the conundrums the lives of these children present to me. Meditation as a means to diagnosis and treatment, did you say? Yes, I did. Meditation is a popular topic these days, though it must be said that if the word itself is not uttered in hushed tones, discussion of its nature and its gifts is often accompanied by overtones of exclusivity. Yet, the Oxford Universal Dictionary defines meditation in very clear, simple and understandable terms. It says meditation is "serious and sustained reflection, or mental contemplation." Contemplation? Alas, another popular topic of the 20th century often swathed in the same garment of exclusivity, as is meditation. But, the same Oxford Dictionary cites it simply as being primarily "attentive consideration and study." Surely, aren't these the very qualities that thoughtful caregivers bring to their charges, and aren't the energies inherent within them basic to human development and evolution, therefore shared by all of humankind despite some current attempts to make of them recently discovered esoteric entities? Within these rubrics, bringing a lifetime of personal experience and professional expertise to bear on the destiny of a child is surely a contemplative meditation, not uncommonly the rewards, like those promised to those who meditate in a more specifically spiritual way, have been for me not only a deeper knowledge of humankind, but also a deeper and immense compassion for its suffering that would not otherwise have been to my knowing. In so many ways, these children and their families have not only been my teachers, but through sharing in their lives, they have become a part of my soul. Thankfully and not infrequently I have in turn become a part of theirs.

On this particular winter's day, my meditative ambiance was abruptly interrupted by the buzz of the intercom. Picking it up, my secretary informed me that Joshua, who was to be the first patient for the afternoon, was delayed and that his social worker was on the line wishing to speak with me. "Please put him through." "Good afternoon, Dr. Anderson," the pleasant voice on the other end of the line said. "I am Nathan Brown, Joshua Seraphim's case worker. I am sorry we are late but last night's storm has made driving conditions very slick. If you can fit us in later this afternoon I would be grateful; otherwise, I will reschedule Joshua's appointment." Knowing how important it was for me to see this child, I replied, "If you are willing to continue the drive, and consider it safe enough to do so, then come on along and I will fit you in." "Thank you, Dr. Anderson, we'll be there in about an hour."

The western part of New York State where I was working that day is known for its great variety of natural beauty. The Niagara River, short in length but mighty in it's marvelous gifts of sight and sound, dominates the region and it, together with Lake Erie from whose waters it takes its life, serve as the western edge of New York State and as part of the geographic boundary between the United States of America and Canada. World famous Niagara Falls, considered one of the seven natural wonders of the world, is where the river falls into a deep cataract on its brief journey between Lake Erie and Lake Ontario, the two most easterly of North Americas five inland Great Lakes. Moving inland, southeast of the Niagara River and the Lakes, the earth of this region burgeons upward into the northern tip of the Appalachian Mountain chain. Running almost parallel to the eastern seaboard, the Appalachian chain extends into the deep South of the U.S. Large tracts of its hills and valleys in Western New York, as indeed, all along the chain have been preserved as state parks, thus providing year-round facilities for recreation and relaxation. In the summer, they offer boundless opportunities for camping, hiking, and fishing and are favorite family vacation spots. In the winter, cold arctic weather systems originating in Canada pick up moisture from the Great Lakes and prevailing winds combined with the right combination of land and lake temperatures can result in extremely heavy falls of snow. Thus, it is no surprise that the mountains of western New York State boast countless beautiful ski resorts, making the area a mecca for ski enthusiasts and other winter sports fans. But, for those who must daily travel to and from work in snow and ice, it is anything but a paradise; indeed, it is often a hazard to be feared.

As I looked out the window that wintry day, I pondered on how the heavy fall of snow, so disarmingly beautiful in its measured persistent fall to earth, would call forth human responses that were polar-opposite and all degrees in-between — a microcosm of the macrocosm that is the response of humankind to life and its many rhythms, like the mirror that each season holds to the human journey. The exuberance of spring and the blossoming of summer, yielding to the magnificence of autumn with its triumphal cry of bounty, beauty, and the color of life well lived, all deriving, not from some capricious act of the gods, but from the memories of past cycles hidden within the secrets and wisdom of its seeds and growth. And then, before the winter, the fall of all to earth. Yet, winter slumber, when all seems dead, is a time that refreshes, replenishes, and gives strength to what lies hidden in the earth so that in the fullness of time the cycle may once again begin. And all is accomplished despite the threats that lurk in each season, ever ready to engage or even to combat survival by disrupting the cycle of growth, of giving and of completion. Through storms, droughts, floods, volcanoes, and even the plunder of humankind, Nature and the soil from which she springs asserts her right *to be* and emerges triumphant, defiantly proclaiming the indestructibility of *Life*. So it is that even in what appears to have been catastrophic destruction such as occurs when volcanoes erupt burning and smothering all vegetation, eventually a flower will emerge through the volcanic ash, then a sapling, some green ground cover, and so on, until the threads of her garments once again clothe the earth with beauty and nourishment for all.

As it is with the earth, so it is with each and every human journey. Though seasons of nature are four, Shakespeare described seven for Man. While no doubt he was using inclusive language, thus including Woman in his reference to Man, ancient wisdom and presently re-emerging beliefs that have lain fallow in the winter of the submergence of feminine spirituality tell us that women, like nature, have four seasons: Birthers, Nurturers, the Wise Older Woman (the Crone), and Death, thus making them perhaps closer relatives to the rhythm of the earth than those of the opposite gender. Through all of these human seasons, as in nature, threats abound, disrupting, interrupting, diminishing, or injuring each experience of their seasons, even abbreviating or abruptly ending the completion of the cycle. Some individuals, regardless of the challenge to survive, be it "dis-ease," accident or loss, will like nature emerge triumphant and assert their right to life. Others will succumb in varying degrees to the events that rob them of their wholeness and well-being.

But, what causes the differences? Is it a function of choice, much like choices that people make in their attitude to the snow — a gift to some, to others a curse? If so, what is at the root of these choices? What prompts and triggers them? Is it something we inherit, something we learn, or even an interplay between the two? Or, is it something we have yet to uncover from the cloaks that presently hide it from our knowing? Could it be all of the above, and, yes, could it be even more than all of this combined?

What follows in this book is a journey that seeks to glimpse the answers to these questions. A bold undertaking for sure. The reader may ask, "Why bother." In this new age of "How To Live" substance and hype there are hundreds of books already begging attention for how to do it and get on with it. And, in the presently prevalent iconoclasm that questions the motives and blemishes the achievements of many, including the saints of our time, who, you may be asking, am I to address these issues?

My answer is twofold. First, if we put this quest into the context of our society, then it is no secret that far from knowing how to live in peace, violence is ripping our world apart. Furthermore, it is no secret that in the normal course of events children become adults and bring to their adulthood behavior, the experiences of their childhoods. Children today are not only victims of violence, but in no small numbers are also perpetrators of it in the battlegrounds of home, neighborhood, and school, as well as in the battlefields of war throughout the world. And, it is no secret either that learning and behavior disorders amongst children in the Western world are already an epidemic.

Surely then something is happening before or within the springtime of the human cycle that threatens, disrupts, and often aborts its summer and autumn. Though often promoted as the cause of violence and nonachievement, the many attempts to redress poverty have done little or nothing to reduce violence, abuse, and neglect or to reverse their fallout once they have been experienced.

Second, based on the Hippocratic Oath to heal and do no harm, my life's work as a physician has brought me insights into the dynamics of these phenomena which, not being within the mainstream of repairing bodily defects in a rather mechanical way, I feel compelled to share, not only with the professionals marching after me whose work it will be to leaven and use them to heal human dysfunction, but more. I wish to invite a humankind that is presently engulfed in confusion to modify and enlarge their concepts of the origins of human mayhem to include the memories, consciousness, and spiritual denouement that is at its center.

My first specialty as physician was Psychiatry, which studies and seeks to adjust disorders of human behavior, these days mostly through the use of drugs. My second was Pediatrics which studies human development and the factors that assail its expected and normal unfoldments. Combine the two and you have a hybrid physician whose joy and privilege it has been to encounter and study the luminous interdependence and constant interaction of our genetic inheritances and inborn tendencies with the circumstances and experiences of our living. So, for over 35 years I have been an observer and a player in the drama that is the interplay of nature and nurture. I have observed how external factors impinge, bombard, modify, mould, and, yes, sometimes twist the human person whose manifestations, as behavior, are then all too often identified as personality. Personality is that upon which, in our ignorance, we often make judgment of others without regard to how it came about. This, then, gives rise to the pernicious habit of creating black and white, good and bad, in our conceptualization of who we and others are. In my clinical work and in my research, I have used the time-honored objective observation and measurement techniques of the Western scientific world. I have, however, also used that precious gift of "sense-ing" and "see-ing" beyond that which is measurable and objective to guide me along the pathways to my understanding and knowing. *Intuition* is the knowing that comes not from the written word, but from that innate ability to synthesize nuances of sensory language and the energy coming from the patient. Intuition is as old as human consciousness and has its roots in the wisdom of our spiritual memory which the scriptures tell us was before all creation. Being difficult to conceptualize and defying precise parameters of definition and measurement, which are the sacred rules of reality in the Western world, it has for too long been dismissed as irrelevant to any study of the human condition. But from its dwelling place in every human soul, it whispers its yearning to touch, to know, and to be known by the world beyond our waking consciousness — the same world that knocks for entrance through our clay shuttered and often narrow doorways begging to reveal to us many of its secrets. All religions invite us to this dialogue. However, in the dualistic ways of Western thinking that for centuries has separated body from soul, it has until recently been disregarded by mainstream medicine to the point where professionals enlightened as to its reality and value have rarely if ever had the courage to discuss this with their peers. Fortunately, this is changing. Intuition is emerging from its closet and is now on its journey to being recognized as a valuable clinical tool and a more accepted constituent of professional counseling.

Within all this experience, and as my understanding of the human cycle grew, it brought me insights into the matrices and textures of the soul, the soil wherein lie our feelings and our emotions, which find their expression in our behavior. It also brought the knowledge that the script written by the memories of all of our experience, even those that flow from generation to generation in our genes, is the tablet upon which we write interpretations of our present experience. And, while this manifests as our particular behavior, it is also both the source of our resilience or of our succumbing to defeat. Fortunately, it is also the tablet upon which we can re-write the script for our living and our lives, thus breaking the consequences of despair and restoring hope to every human spring.

As I reflected on these things, and although I knew few details about the personal history of the child whose arrival I awaited, there could be little doubt as to the basic nature of his problems. Because he had been referred for evaluation and possible therapy due to his acting out and socially unacceptable behavior, his primal problem would be similar to all children with emotional and behavioral problems. Some part of his soul had been injured and probably deeply scarred. To this point in his young life, Joshua's soul, the very essence of whom he really is, had not been immunized against the injuries of his life's experiences. As a consequence, he carried within him a deep sense of disconnectedness from the creative source of his being and he felt alone and abandoned.

To feel and to actually be disconnected from the center of our own being is to endure a profound sense of loss. The universal reaction to loss is grief. Thanks to the pioneering work of Dr. Elizabeth Kubler-Ross in the U.S. and Dr. James Pickering in England, among others, we know that grief calls forth many emotions — denial, anger, depression, and even rage — which anxiously jostle with ideas of how to bargain with powers beyond the merely human for the return of what was lost. Then, and, not infrequently, over an entire lifetime, we gradually accept the inevitable. Whatever may have been the particular loss or losses this child had endured, he plainly was acting out anger, denial, depression, and anxiety in behaviors that were socially disruptive and unacceptable. Of course, it was the behaviors and not the losses and scars on his soul that were the reasons why he was referred. Indeed, a part of his referral stated, "No one could do anything with him." I also knew that unless the confusion within which he existed received a loving and healing intervention, his emotional development would be arrested or hobbled, if not also twisted, resulting in him being permanently emotionally crippled and unable to be in touch with the creative energy at the core of his own being. From this feeling of disconnection would flow a belief that all that was external to him was alien, and therefore to be feared, put down, and even obliterated, thus further crippling his ability to relate to others and to his environment or even to receive from them in an appropriate manner. Cut off from the energies that are life-giving he would, if there were no healing intervention to re-connect him to self and others, develop the only sane way of dealing with such horrendous isolation. Given his age and developmental level, he would in the near future develop a definable psychiatric disorder of a dissocciative nature accompanied by an intensification of his sociopathic behavior. To dissociate means to withdraw. All dissocciative psychiatric disorders, such as so-called schizophrenia, are in my opinion the cry for meaning within one's own being when external reality becomes too painful to endure. Ultimately, without healing for his injured and disconnected soul, his behavior would likely lead to crime and incarceration if not also injury or death to himself and/or others. Pondering these heart-breaking inevitabilities, I knew that moderating the consequences of his soul's injuries, even turning them around, was possible, but certainly *not* through application of current so-called conventional and institutional methods of managing these injured children. These methods have not only failed them, but also society and the world at large. Only by immunizing these children against soul dis-eases and the dysfunctions that flourish from emotional injury and deprivation can their awful consequences of stunted hearts, minds, lives, violence, and crime be prevented. For the umpteenth time I thought how curious it was that, in an age where the marvels of the body's immune system are not only the concerns of scientists and physicians but have become almost a pop-culture fixation, little or no connection has been made between the absence of immunization for the soul and the present pandemic of violence and other human dysfunction.

Before I could conjecture any further, there was a knock on the door. "Come in!" I said. The door opened and in walked Nathan Brown accompanied by Joshua Seraphim. Dragging his feet, as though his boots were filled with lead, shoulders hunched over, head turned downward and to the side, acting more like an old man than a child of 10, Joshua conveyed in his body language and facial expression the weight of the burdens he carried. After he had handed me Joshua's records and the usual greetings and pleasantries had been exchanged, Mr. Brown left Joshua alone with me. At first, uncommunicative and even hostile, Joshua eventually but grudgingly began to flow into and be bathed by the loving, accepting energy I was conveying to him. At first he told me he did not want to see me and that he was not going to talk to me because he just knew it would be all about "that stuff." That *stuff* was about the fact that nobody wanted him, nobody loved him, and nothing could be done about it. His mother had died of cancer when he was one year old. His father had died a few months previously of AIDS. Prior to his illness, Joshua's father had been an uncertain and frequently absent parent. During his illness, weakness and frustration often caused him to physically abuse Joshua, and when his condition had become terminal, he left Joshua in the care of a friend. Joshua had no known siblings. Following the death of his father, Joshua had lived with his only surviving Grandmother for a short time, but she was unable to cope with him and found it necessary to return him to the child-care agency that now wished to place him in foster care. This ten-year-old boy was literally alone and abandoned. As he began to respond to me, he told me he had no feelings, surely a sign of grievous soul injury, and added, "I don't know what love is — it doesn't exist!" followed by, "and if someone does something for you, there's always a catch."

Some twenty to twenty-five minutes into our exchange he reached for one of the family of Teddy Bears I keep in my office. As I watched him touch it, hold it, look at it, and even caress it, I silently said, "Thank goodness!" His sensory pathway of touch was "alive" and responsive. Therefore, with loving hugs and lots of soft toys, we could initiate sending affirming messages to that part of his brain which moderates and controls emotions; perhaps even to the point where we could, through this passive immunization, actually change its chemistry from that which was reinforcing his feelings of abandonment and despair to that which would lift the pall on his life and give him hope. In a litigious society where legitimate concerns for the safety of children have, in some well-publicized instances, escalated into witch-hunts, adults are afraid to touch, let alone hug, children for fear of being charged with assault. For all children, but particularly those most deprived of loving touch and hugs because they are unwanted or have been abandoned, the troubling question is "how" can we give them a sense of being connected to self and others through the stimulation of touch without fear of innocent people being falsely accused of molestation.

Alas, this will never be realized until society in general, and the agencies and professionals who provide "care" to troubled children in particular, becomes aware and accepting of the profound role that touch plays in our lives. The quality of touch experienced around the birthing process, as well as within the first year of life, is pivotal to later behavior because it establishes the fundamental pattern of brain chemistry and its neurotransmitter messenger system that responds to external stimuli. With loving touch, the neurochemical response system is set to perceive and receive lovingly and, in the absence of obvious danger, without fear. When loving touch has been absent or insufficient, the neurochemical response system is set to perceive and receive with caution, if not with suspicion. It therefore perceives danger more often than it actually exists which calls forth increasingly negative and dysfunctional behavioral responses. These escalate with increasing age and more often than not result in psychiatric disorders which are, in fact, sicknesses of the soul. Simply stated, this knowledge adds up to the fact that:

Loving touch is the most powerful immunizing agent of the soul.

Immunology, for all the grandeur it signifies, is simply the presence of a memory that will call forth a protective response toward attack though, of course, it does not protect against attack itself. Thus, when memories within the response system of the soul are set to love and security, the soul becomes immunized with the strength and resilience required to withstand the negative influences and valleys it will traverse during its journey of life. When the response system is deprived of this protective immunization, the soul and its feelings are left wide open to succumb to one or another valley of despair and to the ultimate language of despair which is *violence*.

Immunization against the physically crippling and frequently deadly diseases of childhood is one of the greatest gifts science has rendered humanity in the twentieth century. The development of vaccines, and their increasing usage, has in the Western world done more to reduce childhood morbidity and mortality than any other single factor, surpassing antibiotics and all other drugs in their efficacy.

The general acceptance and utilization of immunization against physical disease is the result not merely of the miracles of microbiology and immunology that have gifted us for over a century and a half. Of equal importance has been the profound changes in belief systems that, until fairly recently, in human history perceived sickness and death as punishments of a wrathful God for the sins and ingratitude of his children. Now, on the threshold of the third millennium, A.D., the extent of the Creator's hand is becoming ever more clear as we learn that health, or its absence, is a mosaic created by the awesome interplay of genetic and environmental energies. Within this equation is the growing belief that each individual can modify, moderate, or change its outcome. While lifestyle, nutrition, and attitude are fundamental ingredients, how to incorporate them in order to exert power in our lives has become a major industry. There is a deluge of self-help books, workshops, audio and visual tapes, movements, etc., chipping away at some part of this whole.

At the present time, however, most, though not all, of this attention is focused on improving physical health. But, we are more than body. Each human being is a trinity of body, mind, and soul whose interplay is constant and continuous. Therefore, the same genetic and environmental factors that impact on bodily health must also combine to form the mosaic at the core of emotional, mental, soul, and spiritual health, as well as their disorders. Similarly, what drives their communicative interplay is the same as it is with the physical body, simply, *Energy*, and energy is amenable to change.

Alas, these concepts, and the use of energy as healer, are presently not a part of the general awareness or therapeutic armamentaria of most health-care providers nor of the insurance companies that hold us hostage to the type of care we can receive. It is, therefore, of little or no surprise that statistics, particularly those pertaining to children with emotional, behavioral and learning disorders, inform us that for the most part current programs of remediation or so called correction are failing soul injured children like Joshua. He is only one of millions of children, another microcosm within a macrocosm who through no fault of their own have been deprived of love and belongingness, as well as the greatest gift of all, *a memory within their soul of having been wanted*. The memory of being wanted from the start is like *loving touch*, a profound immunization of resilience for the soul and it's journey. Failure to truly help these children will continue until we change our present belief systems about the origins of soul disorders, as well as our current practices of treating their emotional and behavioral manifestations. Presently, children like Joshua who are abandoned or in need of security and love are marched through the court systems as though they were criminals. From there they are sent either to foster homes or to residential facilities where too often the behavioral manifestations of their soul distress continues to be disciplined verbally, if not physically, rather than healed spiritually.

We still have far to go in understanding the biology, physiology, and pathology of the soul. But even now we know enough not only to pursue the unraveling of its secrets, but to commit ourselves to ways of preventing or immunizing against the fallout of trauma inflicted on it; we need to tend and nurture the soil of its growth. Eventually, it is to be hoped, immunization of the soul will be as readily accepted as is immunization against physical diseases. If we juxtapose its status today with where it was less than a century and a half ago, we can joyfully expect that the sweet saga of success in control of physical disease can be repeated for diseases of the soul. For what seemed like a dream at that time became a dream come true and how it became so is a thrilling tale. And what does all this mean to Joshua? Well its a long story reaching back perhaps to the dawn of time, so let us begin.

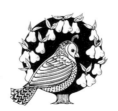

II

The Cry of the Soul to be Immunized

Success of Bodily Immunization

I N JUNE OF 1995, a great benefactor of humankind, and particularly of children, died. His passing was noted by the media, but the full meaning and gift of his life was submerged in the flood of hype that was the coverage of the O.J. Simpson trial.[1] Forty years previously, in 1955, and after many years of dedicated research, it was announced that Dr. Jonas Salk had developed the first vaccine against poliomyelitis. By so doing, he lifted the pall and the fear that lay over the summer months in the Western World for, although always prevalent, the incidence of poliomyelitis peaked in this season. In

---

[1]O.J. Simpson, the former USA football player accused of murdering his former wife, Nicole, and her friend Ronald Goldman.

the U.S. alone between 10,000 to 50,000 individuals, mostly children. were struck down by paralytic poliomyelitis and died or were permanently crippled by it every year. Many more contracted the disease but escaped its deadly and crippling effects. The enormity of Salk's achievement could hardly be measured.

Poliomyelitis had scourged humankind for over a millennia. The earliest recorded evidence of it dates back to the 18th Dynasty of the Egyptian Empire (1580 to 1359 BC). An Egyptian stone relief dating to this period depicts a young priest with an atrophied, shortened leg supporting himself with his staff. Experts believe his deformity was a result of childhood polio. So, not only was Dr. Salk's vaccine a triumph over a scourge that had been present for millennia, it also brought instant hope of protection to millions of people all over the world. As a measure of its success, within six years of its introduction, the incidence of poliomyelitis in the U.S. was reduced by 95% [*Figure 1, Appendix*].

But, his was no easy victory. The methods he used to make his vaccine went against the flow of current beliefs and thus created a controversy that swirled around him until his death. Ironically, shortly thereafter, his beliefs were vindicated. At the eye of the controversy was the fact that as a young scientist, Salk developed his vaccine from viruses that he had subjected to a process of deactivation so that, in effect, he used inactivated or killed viruses. By so doing he challenged the then-held beliefs of the scientific community which contended that all effective vaccines should be made from living organisms. When he asserted that it would not only be safer to use an inactive polio virus, but that it would be just as effective in creating immunity, he was scoffed at and criticized. He conducted his research in the early days of modern immunology when barely a fraction of what is presently known was known then. Yet, even in the context of the enormous knowledge currently available, I believe we are still not fully cognizant of what may ensue from his achievements. His work revolutionized existing theories by demonstrating that the physical immune system is able to create memories of defense against attack when the substance needed to create the memory, which we call the antigen, is changed to the point of being powerless to attack its victim, or is dead. This created a startling and marvelous contradiction and conundrum because in the one, forever certainty of human belief, death has meant total non-responsiveness. By demonstrating that dead material from one phylum of creation could and did interact with living systems of another, in a way that protected life and allowed for its continuance, he unlocked the door to a chest full of treasures many still waiting to be unwrapped. Surely, this interaction must depend on some memory in the dead matter that either is of itself or converts to an energy that can still interact and perform the tasks of the live matter. That this is not only possible, but, in fact, probable flows from one of the great but as yet unappreciated gifts of quantum physics, which is evidence of the interchangeability of matter and energy. Equally tantalizing is the veil that Salk's work drew aside to reveal the persistence of a reactive energy beyond the death of matter. The relation this bears to the power of the memories in the immune system of the soul, from which derive our feelings and behavior, is a vast domain whose territories await exploration in the chapters that follow and from which will emerge the knowledge and the means whereby we can immunize humanity against it's soul dysfunctions.

These are new concepts which will take time to flower. As an example of how difficult it is to let old belief systems die, when eight years after the introduction of the Salk vaccine, Dr. Albert Sabin presented the world with a live polio vaccine in 1963, the ease with which people reverted to old familiar and maybe more comfortable belief systems quickly became apparent. Indeed, it demonstrates well the power of memory on human function and behavior. The Sabin vaccine almost immediately replaced the Salk vaccine and was universally used from that time until very recently. The reasons given for this switch were its ease of administration by mouth, thus avoiding injections, and its lower cost of production. Also, it was thought to enhance immunity by transmission of vaccine viruses to susceptible contacts; thus, serving to immunize them and thus, further limit the spread of naturally occurring polio viruses, but time proved there was a risk.

Poliomyelitis, due to wild, i.e., naturally occurring, or indigenous polio viruses, still occurs in 38% of the 211 countries of the world, but there have been no such cases in the Western hemisphere since 1991. However, there have been eight cases of Sabin live vaccine-associated paralytic poliomyelitis reported annually in the U.S.. Approximately 45% of these cases are recent oral Polio vaccine recipients, mostly infants, and 90% occurred after the first dose. The remaining cases occur among direct contacts of recent live vaccine recipients, mostly siblings, parents, and other family members. Since 1995, wild type polio viruses no longer circulate in the Western world, but so long as they exist elsewhere, the risk of importation must to be considered. Therefore, it will be necessary to continue to immunize children for as long as it takes to eradicate the viruses worldwide — a task, which it is estimated, will take at least another 15 years or more. This means that if the live Sabin vaccine continues to be used, anywhere between 50 to 150 cases of vaccine-induced poliomyelitis may occur annually. Can this be tolerated when in fact the Salk vaccine has never been known to cause the disease? On October 18, 1995, the Advisory Committee on Immunization Practices (ACIP) to the Centers for Disease Control (CDC), which is the world's policeman on these issues, unanimously said, no! In 1997, this same committee gave assent to three schedules that were accepted by the American Academy of Pediatrics and the American Academy of Family Practice and professional organizations elsewhere. The schedules recommended for routine use involve administration of two doses of the now enhanced Salk inactivated polio vaccine (eIPV), followed by two doses of oral polio vaccine. It is believed this will reduce by 50% the frequency of vaccine-associated paralytic poliomyelitis, as well as help facilitate the final transition to an all eIPV schedule of immunization in the U.S. at which time, poliomyelitis due to live vaccine will be eliminated. In Denmark, a similar schedule has been used since 1968 and only one case of live vaccine-associated polio occurred in 1969 in a child who had received only one dose of the Salk vaccine, rather than the three recommended in that country.*

Thus, the far-sighted Dr. Jonas Salk, who 40 years ago challenged the scientific community to change its thinking on how to develop safe as well as effective vaccines, was vindicated. That this vindication came from the community that criticized him, and mostly after his death, is the all too frequent fate of those who truly change the world. However, it must be said that during his life Salk received wide recognition and many accolades from an otherwise grateful world.

Similar success stories exist for all of the presently immunizable diseases, particularly for those to which children are particularly susceptible. For example, in New York City in 1894, the death rate from diphtheria of children aged 10 and under was 785 per 100,000 (785/100,000) children in that age group. In 1920, soon after the development of the diphtheria vaccine and immunization of school children had begun, it fell to less than 100/100,000. Soon thereafter, immunization of preschool children was begun and, by 1940, the death rate for children 10 and under had dropped to 1.1/100,000. Although diphtheria still occurs (*Figure 2, Appendix*), there have been no reported deaths from it, subsequent to national implementation of immunization against it. Figures 3 through 7 (*Appendix*) show how, after introduction of vaccines for whooping cough, tetanus, measles, mumps and rubella (German measles), the incidence of these diseases has dropped dramatically. All of these dis-

---

* In 1999, it was recommended that an all eIPV schedule be used from now on.

eases are similar to polio inasmuch as they tend to cause long-term crippling rather than immediate death. In the case of rubella in pregnant mothers, profound disfiguring and functional defects in their offspring can occur.

As these diseases waned in the face of immunization against them, the occurrence of other less common diseases appeared to rise. Prominent among these were a variety of infections due to a small bacterium named *Hemophilus influenza* which has several siblings and cousins, in particular, one referred to as *type b*. Its greatest menace to infants and children is meningitis, which, if it doesn't kill, leaves heart-breaking and often life-long legacies of blindness, deafness, and other disabilities, a sharp contrast to the suddenness of its onset in previously healthy infants. Before the vaccine for this infection was developed, a question which clinicians often asked of the parent or surrogates of a suddenly seriously ill infant was "When did (s)he last look or smile at you?" If the answer was "over an hour ago," we could be almost certain of the problem and its probable outcome. Thankfully, since the introduction in 1987 of an effective vaccine, the incidence of its invasive disease in infants and children is reported to have declined by 95%.[2] The success of these vaccines has prompted the U.S. Public Health Service to target Hib disease in children younger than 5 years for elimination in the U.S. Its track record in eliminating other killer diseases such as small pox gives hope that this will be accomplished. Additionally it aanounced in January 2000 it was targeting poliomyelitis for elimination worldwide by the year 2001.

Alone among the vaccines presently used, that for whooping cough, often called pertussis after the name of its causative bacterium, is feared by parents because of its reputation for causing adverse reactions, the most serious of which is a condition of shock accom-

---

[2]*Red Book*, 1997; and *Abstract of the 32nd Interscience Conference on Antimicrobial Agents and Chemotherapy*, 1726 (1992).

panied by unresponsiveness. Fortunately, this is a rare occurrence, but, when it happens, it is very alarming. Although follow-up studies on children who suffered these episodes indicate that there are no long-term consequences, nevertheless, research has been underway for some time now to develop a kinder, more reliable vaccine, which has led to new dimensions in our understanding of the intricacies of immunity.[3] Recently, a vaccine developed from products derived from the cells of the pertussis bacterium, but separate from its body, the so-called a-cellular pertussis vaccine has been produced and tested for its immunogenicity in Japan and elsewhere. It appears to confer immunity comparable to the old vaccine that contained the body of the bacterium and it is anticipated that eventually it will replace it. What is fascinating about this development is that I see it as an extension of what Dr. Salk achieved with his inactivated polio virus vaccine which opens the door to rather exciting and profound questions about the nature of immunity itself. Salk's vaccine at least had the "body," although a dead one, of the virus itself. This new acellular vaccine, however, does not contain the body of the pertussis bacterium, dead or alive. If a vaccine can be made without any particulate matter, and is able to create a memory of defense against attack when it is presented to the immune system, then, obviously, energy must be the vehicle of its interaction. If not, then what?[4] Current concepts of how the immune system functions, for the most part stubbornly remain dependent on the interactions that take place between the particulate matter of an attacker and that of the victim, be it even at a level less than molecular. It may be visualized as a series of locks and keys. In other words, if viruses, bacteria, and other thieves of health try to enter the body temple, they must have the key to unlock its defense systems against their particular kind of infection, dysfunction, or disease. But, these acellular

---

[3] *Vaccine Bulletin* (November 1995).

[4] Robert Pool, "Beams of Stuff," *Discover Magazine* (December 1997): 103-107.

vaccines indicate that particulate matter is not required. Rather, it appears as though there is a protective response by the immune system to a resonance presented to it by the vaccine. If resonating frequencies are all that is required for interaction to occur, this takes us to a level of understanding beyond current norms of how the body, mind, and soul interact with each other. It also reveals how sound and light and their many arrangements in music and color are so effective in healing the dissonance of disease and dysfunction.

While all of this awaits further revelation and definition, it is clear that the miracle of immunization has become a *right* and a *rite* of passage for most children. The thoroughness of the protection so conferred is quite evident in the 1998 *Childhood Immunization Schedule* recommended for use in the U.S. which, with minor variations, is replicated throughout the Western world (*Table 1, Appendix*). Yet, it is doubtful if most parents, grandparents, or their surrogates have any knowledge of the origins of these rituals, or of the courage and ingenuity of the few dedicated souls who made it all possible. It is not only a thrilling "whodunit," but it provides powerful lessons on how we may use similar principles to establish vaccines that can be applied to the present killing fields of children which are diseases and dysfunctions of the soul.

For at least a millenium, humans have known that even a tiny dose of a disease agent could confer protection against its otherwise deadly consequences. As early as 900 AD, the Chinese had devised a means for fending off smallpox by inhaling ground-up pox scabs which practice eventually made its way to India and Turkey. But, the real story began with a humble country doctor who lived in England from 1749 to1823. The observations of Dr. Edward Jenner set the stage for the unfolding of a drama that continues to this day. What he observed and put into practice became the infrastructure on which the edifice of immunization was built and upon which the now vast empire of immunology rests. He practiced in the West Country of England — the land of legends and wars, of King

Arthur, Sir Lancelot and Queen Guinevere, and which, during his lifetime, supported an agrarian-centered culture. The observation that opened his way into history was that when people in contact with animals which were infected with cow pox developed the pustules on their own bodies and were subsequently exposed to small pox, they did not develop this deadly disease. The idea that infection with cowpox protected against small pox intrigued him.

To prove the validity of his observations, he conducted an experiment that in today's climate of protection for research subjects would be unthinkable. He inoculated, i.e., injected, a young boy with cowpox matter taken from the hand of an infected milkmaid. Several weeks later he injected the boy with small pox matter. To his delight, and one would hope to his relief, the boy did not develop small pox. Following publication of his findings in 1798, physicians from around the world rushed to reproduce his results. Such was the enthusiasm that in 1800 Dr. Benjamin Waterhouse (1754 to 1840), of Harvard University in the U.S. published an account of his own work with cow pox material sent to him from Dr. Jenner in England. The title of his article was *"A Prospect of Exterminating the Small Pox."* One hundred and seventy years later the U.S. Centers for Disease Control in Atlanta, Georgia proclaimed likewise; this time, however, after a world-wide campaign of vaccination for all people, it stuck and in 1980 small pox was eradicated from the world.

The many paths of inquiry and their fruits unleashed by Dr. Jenner's observations have benefited humankind beyond measure; marvelous though these benefits are, there was in his time no understanding of the underlying mechanisms of how these protective phenomena operated. The first glimmerings in the unraveling of this mystery appeared several decades later. During the mid-to-late 19th century, Louis Pasteur of France, Robert Koch of Germany, Joseph Lister of England, and others, each working independently of the other, demonstrated the role of bacteria and other microorganisms in human disease. This was a watershed in the understanding of human disease. That it would come from several sources simultaneously invites pause to wonder at the synchronicity of thought amongst those following similar paths. Perhaps this is a beautiful example of a particular energy pulsating in the collective consciousness and seeking to bring all of us new awarenesses in our shared journey of evolution. This, indeed, is what happened because their overlapping discoveries allowed for the very first time the cause of sickness to be pinned on something other than weakness or sin within oneself, or even the wrath of God. While this was very liberating, nevertheless, to some extent it may have set the stage for the habits of the mid-to-late 20th century of looking everywhere but within ourselves for our ill health. At the turn of the century, this pendulum appears to be swinging back to center.

The years between 1870 and 1900 saw the dawn of the science of Immunology which is the study of how the human body resists, desists, or succumbs to infection and other disease processes. At first, this was predominantly directed to the study of the body's interaction with micro-organisms. In a broader sense, immunology seeks to inform us of the dynamics involved in the relationship of individuals to their internal and external environments which brings us to a point where, as I have already indicated, we must look more and more to energy and its infinity of wavelengths and their interactions for answers. Nevertheless, over a century ago, Robert Koch in Germany devoted his time and talents to the development of techniques for safe handling of bacteria, thus allowing him to grow pure cultures on which many experiments were made to elucidate more information about them. But as more and more of these organisms were brought to light, and their pathogenic role in human and animal disease confirmed, questions arose regarding the mechanisms of their actions. How did they produce infection? How can infection be prevented? And, how can its consequences be treated?

Starting in about 1871, Louis Pasteur and his associates applied their efforts to finding answers to these questions. From the start, it was obvious from what occurred during epidemics that individual susceptibility and resistance to infection varied considerably. As epidemics of plague, cholera, small pox, and other diseases swept through entire communities, some would succumb while many others who had been in close contact with the victims, would not. So, it appeared that there was something within individuals that modified their response to exposure to infection which, of course, was much later identified as differences in immunity. Meanwhile, logically pursuing his research step-by-step, Pasteur found in laboratory experiments that the virulence of bacterial organisms could be attenuated under various conditions, including exposure to low temperatures. Following the lead of Dr. Jenner, Pasteur conceived the idea of preventing infectious diseases by means of vaccines prepared from these altered or attenuated strains. The successful results of his work on chicken cholera, swine erysipelas, and rabies led to the rapid development of other vaccines, some of which included those for diphtheria, typhoid fever, and tetanus. At about the same time it was also discovered that following administration of vaccines to animals, protective substances appeared in their blood that had therapeutic and prophylactic powers when injected into humans. From these observations, it became clear that immunity against infection could be *actively* generated within a person's own immune system by giving them a vaccine, or it could be *passively* acquired by administration of blood products containing disease-specific antibodies or antitoxins generated in other species.

Though there is little public awareness of how these relatively recent beginnings have brought us to where we are, it is impossible to overemphasize their importance. While improvements in living and social conditions as well as education have had a general overall favorable impact on reducing mortality and morbidity, particularly pertaining to children, no other single entity has had as profound an impact on prevention of childhood sickness as has immunization and the science of immunology that evolved from it. It is hard to believe that despite the wonderful benefits so bestowed, there have been and continue to be those who oppose immunization, mostly on grounds of religious beliefs and fear of infringement of choice and liberty. In the U.S. about 1% of school entrants are exempted from otherwise compulsory immunization because of the religious and philosophical objections of their parents. Debate over the legitimacy of these exemptions led to the formation of a working group to study the issues. Their preliminary findings, submitted in October 1997, indicated that these exemptions do not appear to have a major impact on vaccination rates, but that there impact on possible disease outbreaks needs further study. It was further stated that there were more important areas of child health that should be focused on at this time, a sentiment with which I heartily agree and, none more important than healing the scars on their souls.

The rapidity with which vaccines have evolved is matched only by the brilliance of their success. So much so that in 1993 estimates of the number of children aged 19 to 35 months in the U.S. who were fully immunized, according to the schedule recommended by the Advisory Committee on Immunization Practices of the Centers for Disease Control, was the highest ever reported. Even so, it was also estimated that approximately 2 million children 2 years of age and under lacked one or more of the recommended doses, particularly for *Haemophilus influenza b* and *Hepatitis B*. This high level of population immunization was unprecedented. Nevertheless, on October 1, 1994 the U.S. federal government enacted the *Vaccines for Children Program* and appropriated $1 billion to implement it. The Act was intended to provide free vaccines for children aged 18 and under who were eligible for federally funded health programs. Also included were those not having health insurance or whose insurance would not cover vaccines. The overall objective was to achieve complete immunization for 90% of 2 year olds by the year

2000 AD.[5] Given that many children in these groups do not receive adequate health supervision, it was argued, on what grounds remains a mystery, that the Vaccine for Children program (VFC) would enable more children to receive health care through their primary physician and that they would be immunized on time. This is an assumption that bears no relation to the well-documented behavioral patterns of those it is intended to benefit, plus the fact that most of these children do not have a primary physician. From the outset, the bill had vociferous opponents on the grounds that it was redundant, and after a year of operation, it was found to have had very little impact on population groups with previously low immunization rates. The words of one health official echo many others: "We have enough vaccine and have no problem with distribution. What we do not have is enough nurses to give it, clerical staff to track it, and outreach workers to bring them in."[6] Without providing these and other ingredients necessary to heighten the awareness of parents or their surrogates to the necessity for children to receive regular health care and supervision, as well as immunizations, nothing will change.[7] And this, as we shall discover, is at the core of the disease and dysfunction that presently cripple and kill our children.

Several studies have demonstrated that children who are under-immunized also make substantially fewer preventive health care visits as well as fewer illness visits to any health care facility, let alone a primary care physician. Quite obviously they and their caretakers have minimal contact with the healthcare system.[8] In an article in

---

[5]*Vaccine Bulletin* (November 1995).

[6]*Vaccine Bulletin* (September 1995).

[7]Carole Lannon et al., "What Mothers Say About Why Poor Children Fall Behind in Immunizations," *Archives of Pediatrics and Adolescent Medicine*, 149 (October 1995).

[8]Lance Rodewald et al., *Archives of Pediatric and Adolescent Medicine*, 149 (October 1995): 393-95.

the October 1997 issue of *Archives of Pediatrics and Adolescent Medicine*, the researchers stated that just providing free vaccines in a barrier-free system will not ensure the 90% immunization levels hoped for by 2000 AD for children aged 2 and under. Not surprisingly, they concluded that continuity of care was the vital ingredient and that most of the population they studied who had received a full series of vaccines by the age of two were in some situation where this was a factor including those children who attended day care.

Continuity and comprehensiveness of care have for decades now been considered the lynch-pins of adequate health and medical care not only for children but the entire population, and the medical and social literature dating back as far as 35 years ago is full of references to their importance. Rediscovering them as essential components to the success of any national health initiative is in line with what appears to be an era of rediscovery of important issues, which had they been initially addressed, would have produced a landscape far different from what we presently have. For example, recent articles have highlighted the importance of early detection of deafness in infants and of the ongoing need to detect hearing loss, but there is ample evidence that these concerns have been very well addressed and repetitively so over the past 50 years. Nevertheless, as a measure of what can be achieved when the national will is applied to solving such problems, the U.S. Centers for Disease Control reported that as a result of the tremendous focus put on immunization by the Vaccines for Children program, vaccination coverage in 1996 increased significantly from the baseline year of 1992 from 83 to 95% for three or more doses of DPT; from 72 to 91% for three or more doses of Polio vaccine; from 28% to a whopping 92% for three or more doses of *Haemophilus influenza* type B (Hib); and from 8 to 82% for coverage with three or more doses of *Hepatitis B* vaccine. The recent advent of DNA vaccination technology promises to revolutionize the practice of human immunization. It differs from traditional vaccines in that just the DNA cod-

ing for a specific component of a disease-causing organism is injected into the body. Traditional vaccine development strategies do not
work on some pathogens, one notable example being malaria, but
using DNA vaccination technology, a promising vaccine candidate
has been developed for malaria and for 15 other human illnesses.
While much further research is still required, nevertheless, it is possible that DNA vaccines and other new methods, including transcutaneous and edible forms, may in the foreseeable future make
individual and community protection against many communicable
diseases a relatively easy goal to attain, always providing there is a
viable public health network to promote and support it. The recent
extensive restructuring in the health care sector, with its present
emphasis on insurance and payment mechanisms rather than the
prevention and treatment of disease, has pushed public health activities and their proven worth to society almost into oblivion. But the
findings of two recent surveys, one conducted nationally and the
other in California, indicate significant support for public health
services and strongly suggest a need for further definition of its
legitimate activities.[9] This takes on great significance when put into
the context of the current spectrum of childhood morbidity whose
causes and fallout affect all of society everywhere in the world. The
causes are abuse and neglect deriving from lack of respect for the
dignity of the child; the fallout grasps the pain of lost childhoods
and the broken and often violent lives of the adults they become.
Yet, neither of these surveys asked a single question about this
worldwide epidemic.

Over the years, epidemiologists, who are the professionals who
know all about the "ins" and "outs" of disease as it relates to popu-
lations, have calculated what percentage of the population must be
immunized in order to eradicate certain infections. This is referred

---

[9]*MMWR*, 474 (1998):69-73; Vaccine Bulletin 115 (May 1998); and Hepatitis
Weekly (December 15, 1997).

too as "herd" immunity. Table 2 (*Appendix*) lists these percentages for a variety of viral, bacterial, and protozoan infections in developed and developing countries. Tables 3 (*Appendix*) shows the percentage of children entering school in the U.S. who are fully immunized against diphtheria, pertussis, tetanus, poliomyelitis, mumps, measles and rubella for the years 1980 to 1993. By comparing these two tables, it is obvious that by the time they enter school, the immunization levels of children for these diseases exceeded those required for herd immunity.

Yet, every 75 minutes a child in the U.S. is starved, beaten, shot or killed in some violent manner. Alarmingly, it has become the case that sometimes a child does the beating, shooting, and killing. Occasional wife battery is estimated to exist in 16% of families and 3.4%, i.e., 1.8 million women, are beaten regularly by their partners. In one study, 40% of mothers interviewed reported that in their families violence was used as a means to "settle" disagreements. In 1985, a National Family Violence Study revealed that more than 3.3 million children per year witnessed physical assault between their parents.[10] A study done at the Pediatric Primary Care Clinic at Boston City Hospital reported that 10% of the children treated there had witnessed shootings or stabbings before the age of 6 years, and half occurred at home. In Los Angeles County, the Sheriff's Sexual Assault investigators estimated that a child is present in 50% of rapes occurring at home.[11] These are the memories that too many children are carrying throughout their lives — memories that, once having taken root in their souls, are all too frequently expressed as their own dysfunctional behavior.

---

[10]M.A. Strauss and R.J. Gelles, "How Violent Are American Families," in *Family Abuse and its Consequences: New Directions in Research* (Beverly Hills, CA: Sage Publications, 1988); and Gelles, *Family Violence* (Newbury Park, CA: Sage Publications, 1987).

[11]*Pediatrics*, 96, 3 (September 1995).

There are, as yet, no clinical or population levels established for herd immunity against violence; yet children are being emotionally and spiritually crippled by it, and not infrequently dying of it and society is suffering from it. It is a contagion being passed from generation to generation. We talk about it as a full-blown disease, yet we treat it with the bandaids available through the legal system, through incarceration, parole and other means, all of which too often deepen the wounds that cause it.

Table 4 (*Appendix*) shows the number of cases of each of the immunizable diseases for children aged 5 and under for the year 1994. Table 5 (*Appendix*), which is the most recent data available, shows the number of children reported as victims of neglect and abuse during 1993 and 1994. Not included are those who were not reported, as well as the millions of children who daily suffered withering, soul-destroying, verbal and emotional abuse from parents and/or family members. Though we would like to have seen zero cases of vaccine-preventable diseases, nevertheless, their numbers are few, all except for whooping cough, but even this was less than 300. Yet, in the same time frame, there were almost 3 million children investigated by child protection agencies following reports of suspected abuse and/or neglect, and over another 1 million were dealt with in the juvenile courts (Table 6, Appendix). As a measure of the despair of young people, Table 7 shows the number of delinquency cases disposed by juvenile courts for the years 1983 to 1993. A recent heart-warming development in this regard is the involvement of teens themselves in overcoming the despair and sense of hopelessness experienced by so many of them and which too often leads to suicide. In Toronto, Canada, students have founded a group named "Students Against Violation of Life" (SAVOL). In May 1999, they organized a dance to raise money to provide counseling services to those of their number who required counseling. Bravo! for these fine young people.

The statistics speak for themselves. The disparity between

where our efforts are being directed and where they should be directed leaves one speechless. Why, one must ask, is money, effort, and emphasis being placed on and in programs for what essentially is *not* a problem, while the real problems are left to take their toll? Could it be that we flounder because we do not know what to do and maybe feel overwhelmed by its magnitude? I believe this is part of the answer, but at its center is a dissonance between the problems themselves and the coping strategies we presently employ which are failing. Obviously, our belief systems about the causes and management of these soul dysfunctions are in desperate need of revision.

The feelings within our souls from which derive our behavior take their life and sustenance from the memories in our many-layered consciousness. Prior to the discoveries that led to immunization against infectious diseases, the microbial organisms that caused them worked their invasiveness and destruction from memories of how to do so stored in their genetic and cellular material and passed through numberless generations of their kind. The success stories of immunization inform us of what is possible when destructive memories can no longer operate due to defenses created against them. If human behavior is beholden to memories in the soul likewise passed from generation to generation, then the statistics that describe the appalling extent of child abuse and neglect reflect an equally appalling sickness of the collective human soul. We need to lighten this darkness by finding ways to immunize the soul, and because memories drive it, then it behooves us to find ways to change or modify those that are destructive for present and future generations. In this regard, I believe we are at a stage similar to that of over a century ago when Pasteur, Koch, Lister, and others stood on the threshold of their discoveries, the fruits of which we now take for granted.

As we start on this journey of discovery and healing, our map will be similar to that used by Pasteur when seeking answers to the questions he asked when pursuing vaccines for physical diseases. So we will seek the sources of soul dysfunction and the matrices of its symptoms. From here, we will travel to the territories of prevention and treatment of its consequences. Along the way, we will encounter many junctures of change that will lead us to new horizons of human function and potential. We will discover that memory and consciousness are constant fellow travelers in our pilgrimage and that energy is sustenance to both. To enable us to better traverse the territories of exploration, our first stop on this journey will be at a place called immunity and its environs which reside within the township of Immunology.

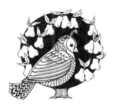

III

The Place Called Immunity and the Township of Immunology

S INCE THE TIME OF THE PERSON of Job, whose life and sufferings are recorded and scrutinized in the Hebrew scriptures, and no doubt reaching far beyond him into unrecorded antiquity, humankind has railed against the capriciousness of nature and it's sometimes destructive intrusion in their lives. Until this present day, natural disasters, while still escaping a full understanding of their cause and ways to contain the damage they wreak, nevertheless, in the past appeared to be in collusion with unseen forces that seemed to arbitrarily choose the sites of their visitations. So it also was with the plagues and epidemics that marched through history. Sweeping through villages, towns, and countryside alike, there appeared to be selectivity in who was affected. No wonder that superstition grew like weeds around marauders who could take one family, leave the one next door, and, above all, indulge preference for children.

In his anguish Job, the good man, at first, railed against a God who could so afflict him by taking all that he was and had for what appeared to be no good or valid reason. His cries of confusion and despair have echoed throughout the ages. Countless multitudes of people who have themselves or whose loved ones have been afflicted by disease or misfortune have in their anguish cried the self-same questions: "Why me? What have I done to deserve this terrible fate?" In these situations, the natural inclination of most is to search their memory for that which they did or did not do and of a dimension great enough to be perceived by God as equitable punishment for their suffering. Indeed, in the extremity of his suffering and before he uttered the words that reflected his awareness that what was given as gift could be taken away, Job asked his God, "What are you remembering about my life — what I did or did not do, which I do not remember, that you should so afflict me?" Though he received no immediate or audible answer, in fact, his question was of the very essence of whom he was and how he came to be. What God was remembering is what humankind is in the infancy of discovering namely, that at the center of all human existence, indeed, of all creation, is memory and its infinity of expression.

The fruits of memory's seeds are passed from generation to generation by way of both energy and matter. Their expression is modified, maybe even altered, by the nature and texture of the soil in which the seeds are planted and the environment in which they must subsequently grow and develop. This soil, and this environment, is CONSCIOUSNESS: personal, transgenerational, and collective. Yet, as if to prove the interdependence of all of life's experiences and how each plays a part in the mosaic of knowledge, it was from out of the decimation wrought by infections that the saga of memory and its many roles and functions in the immune system of the human body began to unfold. Taking the gifts of our existence for granted as we so often do, nevertheless, one has to wonder at the source of the brilliant inspiration that prompted Louis Pasteur as well as others, to simultaneously conduct the experiments that led to the development of vaccines. It could be, and most likely is a perfect example of a common thought seeking expression through more than one mind at particular points in the evolution of humankind. The scientific and spiritual parameters of these kind of phenomena are currently receiving wide attention. No doubt they spring from a deep level of collective consciousness and the energy that drives it, somewhat similar to the singular inspiration of others, like Einstein, who, in his reveries saw waves of energy in patterns from which in his waking consciousness he developed the famous formula $E = MC^2$. From this formula emerged an invitation to humankind to perceive energy, rather than the atom and its particulate components and descendents, as the basis and infrastructure of *life*, an invitation to which many have yet to respond. *Energy* — with its elusive content and myriad wave patterns — still puzzles us in terms of its role in human physiology and pathology but with accelerating intensity it is taking scientists down many avenues of research in quest of the secrets of creation. From the beginning of time, *change*, particularly in belief systems, has always been attended by resistance and skeptics. Pasteur's works and theories, as well as those of Koch, Lister, and others were no exception. Despite the overwhelming evidence that microbial organisms caused infectious diseases, there were some scientists who vigorously opposed this possibility. Speaking at the first meeting of the American Public Health Association in 1873, the President of Columbia College in New York City, F.A.P. Barnard, stated, "If these doctrines of germ theory and evolution are true then all creation becomes absurdity ... if this after all is the best that science can give me then, I pray, no

---

[1]F.A.P. Bernard, "The Germ Theory of Disease and Its Relation to Hygiene." *Public Health Papers and Reports of the American Public Health Association*, 1 (1873): 80-97.

more science."[1] Such strong and scathing language reflects the extent to which Pasteur was challenging hitherto commonly held beliefs, even though he had incontrovertible proof for the truth of what he was saying. The source and energies that led him to his discoveries, and the experiments that preceded them, were not only great intellect and powers of reasoning, but no doubt, in no small measure` that which also guided Einstein and others who have changed the history of humankind, namely, the wordless insights of intuition – the genie and genius quietly at work within our consciousness. If disengaged from the restrictive fetters of our waking conscious and controlling thoughts, intuition never fails to render gifts whose descriptions at first lie beyond the confines of language. It is the high drama of which the poet William Blake spoke when he wrote, "If the doors of perception were cleansed, everything would appear to humankind as it is ... Infinite."

The door that opened to the science of immunology was Pasteur's discovery that external influences could change the behavior of microbes and their interactions with humans and animals. It was the first step to our understanding of how the human immune system operates and of how the memories in the genes make for differences among individuals that, in affliction, leads humanity, as it led Job, to ask, "Why me?" It raised endless questions, many still unanswered, about the intrinsic nature of microbes as well as their relationships to humans and animals in both their natural and attenuated forms. From the start, it was obvious that these were not fixed equations. On the contrary, they were given to many variations and apparently subject to change. By the turn of the 20th century in the Western world, focused inquiry into the forces operating in these equations, as well as their modus operandi, became the lynch-pin of medical research and remained so for several decades. The knowledge so gained became the infrastructure upon which all immunization programs were built and ultimately it provided the ignition to the science of immunology. Yet, within all of this wealth, an intriguing mystery is, how little attention was given to exploring, let alone defining, the mechanisms involved in the attenuation of microorganisms. It appears as if this question was trampled on and then forgotten in what understandably was the headlong rush to develop vaccines from attenuated strains. Yet, attenuation of their power to destroy was and is at the heart of the control of infectious disease. It is by administering small and measured doses of attenuated organisms that the immune system is able to create memories of defense against future attack by unattenuated strains that otherwise would lead to serious illness or even death. Perhaps the enormity of such an undertaking, as well as the unavailability of equipment that would permit it, created the vacuum. But, as often happens in the affairs of humankind, light is shed on buried treasure from unexpected sources and sometimes from apparently unconnected phenomena awaiting intuition and perception to yet again make the connection. Though I am not aware of it being referred to in the scientific literature, I believe the dynamics of attenuation can be extrapolated from the findings of the research on the structure of genes and its application to gene therapy. This, of course, is of very recent origin. It began in earnest following the discovery by Dr. Crick and Dr. Watson in 1965 of the double helix structure of deoxyribonucleic acid (DNA). We know that these helices are exquisitely arranged in a manner that allows their messages of form and function to be conveyed to cellular and transcellular activities where they are implemented. These messages are conveyed through the electrochemical and energy systems of our minds and bodies to every living cell and its component parts. Moreover, when the time comes for reproduction of the species, the form and function of the next generation is conveyed through the messages contained within the genes of the parents.

The centerpiece in the accurate conveyance of messages is MEMORY. So finely tuned are the memories in our genes that when even one molecule gets misplaced or displaced in one gene, it not only causes dysfunction of its specific function but it can also have a domino effect on the whole organism or person — resulting in mild to catastrophic illness and/or crippling. When these faulty but non-lethal memories are passed from generation to generation, we call their effects genetically determined disease. When it happens apparently spontaneously, we call it a genetic mutation. No doubt, in time, we will learn that mutation is a response to a noxious stimulus that may have gone completely unnoticed. It should be noted that many genetically determined diseases originated in a genetic mutation designed to protect the individual against external hazards. Such a case is that of sickle-cell anemia. In Africa, where the malaria parasite was omnipresent, the red blood cells changed their shape to make it more difficult for the malaria parasites to penetrate them, thus providing protection to the individual through increased resistance to infection by them. However, generations later, in a different and relatively malaria-free environment, the altered shape of the red blood cells frequently caused them to disintegrate, leading to breakdown of red cells which then can clog the circulatory system in various locations of the body leading to shock and sometimes death. Such episodes are called hemolytic crises.

Starting in the late 1980s, and armed with their new-found knowledge of gene structure, scientists took off like rockets to find the utopia of a world freed from genetically determined diseases. Their purpose was to supplant defective genes with their normal counterparts. This process was named genetic engineering. In effect, what is intended to take place is replacement of the scrambled incorrect messages from the faulty memory of the damaged gene with correct messages from the restored memory of the normal gene, thus restoring normal function and eliminating dysfunction and disease.

Genetic engineering is in its infancy and so far is actively challenging preconceived notions and paradigms of how it should work. Nevertheless, I believe that what takes place in the process of attenuation of microbial organisms is, in fact, a feat of very simple genetic engineering. What occurs is an intrusion into and subsequent alteration of specific operational memory systems of the microorganism. These operational memories are, in essence, the blueprints and instructions developed and modified over centuries of contact with humans and animals as to how to attack and where to attack their victims so as to overcome them, thus assuring the continuance of their strains through survival and reproduction. They involve, therefore, both functional and behavioral memories and they reside within identifiable components of the organisms which are called antigens. When attenuated, the operational attack memories are modified either because they lose normal patterns and sequences of DNA and RNA within their antigenic memories of attack or because the energies that drive them are changed. Therefore, instead of attacking their hosts, they behave as protectors by allowing the victim's immune system to manufacture substances called antibodies and antitoxins that provide present and future defense against similar attack. In other words, the individual becomes immune to the disease, allowing peace to be made between attacker and attacked. Furthermore, not only are their memories of function and behavior altered, so, too, are their memories of form. When subjected to suboptimal growing conditions in the laboratory, colonies of virulent strains lose their smooth form and become rough-edged colonies. In addition, they lose strength. It is as though, once domesticated in the laboratory, they settle into a cozy life. Nurturing themselves from the nutrients in the culture medium in which they are grown, they no longer have to seek a victim in which to grow and reproduce as they do in their natural wild state. Surely, this demonstrates in a profound way the equality of "nature and nurture," whose interplay has been obscured by the tenets of 20th century sociology and their emphasis on nurture. But, though observable form, function, and behavior have been changed, something essential to the identity of the organism has remained unchanged which allows it to engage its host. What is interesting, if not fascinating for its possibilities when applied to other interactions and functions, is that this process can be reversed and their behavioral memories of attack can be reestablished. While not being absolute proof, nevertheless, this is strongly suggestive that nonparticulate energy is the vehicle whereby the antigen operates, and by attenuating, it's wavelength and/or wave pattern, its memories and therefore its behavior can be altered. If we extrapolate this phenomenon to the functions of mind and soul then, if memory is at the center of our lives, and indeed of whom we are, and if it operates through transmission of energies whose wave lengths and patterns can be altered, then the implications for the understanding management and healing of the memories that underlie emotional and behavioral disorders is profound.

That energy, rather than just the interactions of particles without their energies, is at the center of life is reinforced by an article in the February 1996 issue of Science. In 1994, scientists were jubilant when they discovered the sixth quark, the finest subatomic particle – the bottom line as it were in nature's building blocks. Now they are not so jubilant because it is believed that there is something else lurking in nature's tiniest particle. Surely, this must be enigmatic energy. If so, then subatomic physics may become a lot more interesting because the current standard model of atoms and their progeny as fixed structures of matter will have to be fundamentally revised. So, also, will many of our current concepts of human physiology and its pathology.

All of this is, of course, just the cutting edge to what was and is yet to come. However, it is a far cry from the days not too long ago when those who wrestled with the secrets of creation and sought answers to the causes of human suffering were in danger of their lives. History tells us of the dangers faced by Galileo and many others who dared to question the status quo as well as those who controlled it and believed these were God's secrets, not to be tampered with. Indeed, when Job asked God, "Why do you oppose and afflict me?" God did not respond but instead challenged him by asking, "Where were you when I founded the earth, and who are you to obscure divine plans with words of ignorance?" Such reproof is open to interpretation and could be used as reason to stifle inquiry. But, it can also be interpreted as the call of God to humankind to stop obscuring God and divine plans with words flowing from human ignorance. Most ignorance derives from long-held belief systems that actually emerged from the darkness of superstition and prejudice. Therefore, we owe much to those brave souls who, despite opposition and danger, responded to this call of inquiry and exploration which has brought all of us to new thresholds of understanding the awesome intricacies of life. Not least amongst these pioneers are those who began to unravel the mystery and the majesty of how we humans co-exist, survive, grow, and evolve despite the thrusts from the rest of creation that would have us cry "uncle" and succumb to them.

From its beginnings in the development of vaccines, the science of immunology has traced a meteoric trajectory through all of the biological and behavioral sciences and is still reaching for its outer limits. But prior to this, glimmers of how immunity operates arrived with the dawn of the 20th century and the work of great pioneers such as Metchinkoff, Wright, and others who gave the world its first photographs of the interactions that take place between microbial agents and their hosts. They chose to call the primary reaction of the body to infection, "inflammation." Derived from the Latin, *inflammare*, its original meaning referred to a condition of being "in flames" or of being "set on fire." This describes well what can be seen in external infections, namely, excessive heat, swelling, and redness, which is accompanied by pain. With the assistance of early microscopes, it was possible to demonstrate for the first time what was going on behind the scenes perceived with the naked eye. From these observations, it became apparent that following invasion of body tissues by microorganisms, white blood cells (WBCs) rushed in large numbers to the affected area. It was deduced, and correctly so, that signals were sent from the affected area to the body's reservoirs of WBCs. Then, with the assistance of substances in the blood plasma, called humoral antibodies, the white blood cells attack and disarm the organism and prepare them for ingestion and subsequent digestion by other cells in the blood which are called phagocytes of which there are several types. If the mission is successful, the WBCs and other assistants who survived the combat return to their stations in various parts of the body. If the infection is not contained to the original site and spreads to other parts of the body, the procedures of defense are replicated until the battle is won, health and the status quo are restored, or the host is overwhelmed and succumbs to the effects of the microbial invasion.

These activities are very similar to what takes place when insects are caught in a spider's web. One evening last summer I was sitting on the porch of my home enjoying the peace and beauty of the sunset. A hornet had been buzzing around me for several minutes. Not wanting to swat it, I let it continue along with its evening rituals. Suddenly the buzzing stopped. The hornet had landed at the bottom of the railing on the porch and, upon closer inspection, I saw that it was caught on the edge of a spider's web. Then, out of nowhere, I noticed the spider descending rapidly from the upper part of the web on its way to encounter its visitor. It visited only for a fraction of a second and than instantly returned from whence it came. Meanwhile, the hornet became still and a few hours later I found its remains, its hard outer coat still entangled but now in bits throughout the web. Its succulent parts were, no doubt, now a part of the spider!

How did the spider know that something was caught in the outermost part of the web? What did it do to immobilize its prey? Why was it so confident of the outcome of its actions that it immediately returned to its task of web-weaving at a distance away? In addition, why did the hornet succumb so rapidly while other insects would not in the first place be caught hovering near a spider's web let alone be caught dead in one? Obviously, these events, as in inflammation, derive from the intricate messenger system that has been conditioned to respond to certain stimuli. Since not all stimuli evoke the response, the nature or character of the stimulus itself must somehow be retained in a similar or parallel memory system to which it responds. Clarification of these phenomena rests within knowledge gained over the last three decades from research in human immunology and lately, in that vast arena of psycho-neuro immunology, where once many disciplines resided, but whose future, depending on one's point of view, is said to be at a cross-roads. In an interesting critique of its present status, Dr. Ruth Lloyd, author of *Explorations in Psycho-Neuro Immunology*, argues that a new direction can only come from a theoretical formulation that would temper the strongly reductionist bias that has thus far dominated the scene.[2] However, in general, we know that the behavioral responses of the immune system to external threats are encoded in a precise order of progression from one task to the next. This encoding is not only species-specific but, at some point in this cascade of events, unique to each individual — and these differences are genetically determined, meaning they are memories within our genes.

So, not only are we identifiable by our fingerprints, but also by our DNA and markers in our immune systems. However, for there to be an interaction between attacker and the attacked, they must share somewhere in their messenger systems a means of recognition through and by which their engagement can take place. This is the *deja vu* of transgenerational memory that resides within each of them and which itself derives from countless encounters between their respective ancestors. These encounters have themselves been

---

[2]Ruth Lloyd, "New Directions: Psycho-Neuro Immunology, A Critique." *Advances*, 12, 1 (1990).

modified throughout time by environmental factors that altered the rhythm and nature of their expression. This is why, although microorganisms are always present, except of course for those of small pox which have been eliminated, epidemics caused by one or the other of them come and go.* All of this sets the stage upon which the dance of immunology can be performed. The messages and responses are themselves mediated as, indeed, they are throughout nature and in all functions of body mind and soul by electrochemical and other energy means.

For several decades following the initial description of what took place in inflammation, little further progress was made until the arrival of the antibiotic era. Their almost universal usage in the Western world by the 1960s, and their spectacular ability to fight infections gave a jump-start of sorts to research into the next level of our understanding about immunity and immunology. It was discovered that some antibiotics acted like riot policemen, preventing multiplication of the bacteria causing the infection. By competing with them for access to the cellular substances of the host needed by the microorganisms for survival and multiplication, they serve notice on them to cease and desist from attack. In other words, they put up a large stop sign and thus the nature of their action is termed "bacteriostatic." The host's immune system is then left with the job of clean up and repairs. Examples of such bacteriostatic antibiotics are the sulfonamides, erythromycin, and the tetracyclines. Others act like gangbusters, actually engaging the microorganisms and killing them. Being killers, the nature of their actions is called "bacteriocidal." Examples are the extended family of penicillins and the several generations of cephalosporins. Whether bacteriostatic or bacteriocidal, quite obviously in the presence of microorganisms, they initiate a struggle for control of the host – a struggle in which the immune system of the host is more than just an interested bystander. While the antibiotics are fighting their battles, the

---

*Eliminated from *circulation*, but some are retained in laboratories world wide.

immune system is entering into its memory data bank details of the attacker — thus, building its own defenses against further assaults from the attacker. The immune system also does the mopping up jobs, which enables tissues and hosts to return to a state of health. Its central and essential role is emphasized by the relapses that can occur after administration of antibiotics when, for whatever reason, the immune system is in a weakened state or when the amount of antibiotics administered is insufficient for the virulence and aggressiveness of the bacteria. This brings us to the crucial understanding that, in the final analysis, it is the trinity of body, mind, and soul that heals itself, and all else are merely tools to bring this about.

The popular conceptualization of how the physical immune system functions derives from our knowledge of what occurs when it is fighting off disease and infection in high gear, but, in fact, it never sleeps. The immune system's response capabilities rival those of the nervous system; however, it operates under fewer constraints, befitting the nature of its defensive functions and the fact that it has no fixed architecture. Although it is not inaccurate to state that the immune system is everywhere in the body, its most numerous anatomical sites are the lymph nodes that lie along the lymphatic drainage system throughout the body. Other centers are the thymus gland, the spleen, tonsils, adenoids, appendix, Peyer's patches in the small intestine, and the marrow of long bones. It is constantly on patrol, identifying foreigners such as bacteria, viruses, and abnormal material such as cancer cells and damaged tissue that it recognizes as being *not-self*. It then eliminates them. It fulfills its role in several ways that for simplification may be conceived as two interrelated mechanisms: cellular immunity and humoral immunity.

Cellular immunity is mediated by several subclasses of white blood cells, also known as lymphocytes. These act either directly on the invader or by secretion of chemical mediators called lymphokines, which among other actions activate phagocytes, the host's scavenger cells that destroy their attackers.

The function of humoral immunity relies on a class of proteins called antibodies. They are secreted into the blood by plasma cells, another sub-class of lymphocytes, and then circulate independently.

Messages that pass between the multitude of cellular and humoral elements in the immune system must do so with the speed of light or sound which gives rise to brief but powerful interactions in the blood and lymphatic tissues. Central to the accurate functioning of the immune system, as, indeed, in all systems of the body, is memory: memory that recognizes all that is non-self and defends against it — thus, protecting self. Should it falter, or make a mistake between self and non-self, it could and would consume the individual it is supposed to protect. This is precisely what happens in the so-called autoimmune diseases, of which rheumatoid arthritis is an example. In these conditions a stimulus mobilizes the immunological defense systems in an inflammatory reaction, but, unlike the normal inflammatory response wherein the involved components recede into a normal but watchful state following its resolution, the inflammatory process continues unabated. This chronic inflammation results in destruction of body tissues and systemic illness. Although our knowledge of the immune system has far to go, nevertheless, we do know that the first step in the dance that is immunity comes from a pulse of recognition.

In some degree, it is similar to the manner by which locks and keys work. If the key fits the lock, entrance is permitted, and all is well. If it does not, then the immune system mobilizes its functions of defense. In the combat that ensues, the adversary is trying to adjust its key to the lock it wishes to turn, and the immune system is resisting its efforts. However, in so doing, it is also as it were taking notes as to the form and structure of the key that its adversary is using. Filing these notes in its memory bank, it then builds up immunity against further attack as it manufactures resistance to the keys, which it does by altering slightly the lock that the intruder is attempting to spring. Moreover, as with all locks and keys, there are countless varieties of locks as well as a vast array of entities all busy adjusting their keys in order to enter. Though there is a fundamental and commonly shared pattern to this system of locks that protect the body temple, there are differences that in aggregate render each unique and specific to the individual. Some are protective, conferring increased resistance, while others cause increased vulnerability. Many of these differences are genetic in origin — their memories having been passed from generation to generation — memories that are susceptible to modification by the experiences and environment in which they reside at any particular time. If this happens in the body, does it not also happen in the soul, which is the repository of our feelings, which in turn are the parents of our behavior? When feelings are injured, scars remain whose memories serve to cast shadows across the soul's connection to the source of its life in God and creation, for soul, like body, functions from many layers of memory.

Immunity is all about the preservation of *self*. When *self* is damaged by feelings of disconnection, we lose our identity and *non-self* takes over. The resulting confusion gives rise to disordered thought processes and dysfunctional behaviors, both of which are inherent components of all psychiatric disorders. It is not hard to understand how, if *non-self* is dominant, the true personality of the individual will be submerged. This damaged sense of *self* is, I believe, at the root of all personality disorders as well as at the center of the so-called dissociative psychoses.

Thus, if we are to address the real healing of psychiatric disorders and their terrible fall-out on individuals, families, and nations, we must find ways of immunizing the soul.

Since immunity is based on memory and its offspring of recognition and discrimination, our first endeavor must be to attain a deeper understanding of how memory works its ways in our life.

However, before we continue on this journey of exploration,

can we, at the dawn of the 21st century, with the knowledge we presently have answer Job's question to God? "What are you remembering about me and my life, that I do not remember, that you should so afflict me?"[2] What the all-knowing God knew was Job's own unique immune system and the mismatch of some of its keys and locks. And for the condition itself? Two alternatives are possible. An overwhelming infection that eventually itself was overwhelmed by the response of his immune system or an autoimmune disease that went into remission as these diseases often do. That it was the latter is suggested by the timing of his recovery. It occurred when he stopped railing against his misfortunes and, in accepting them, found and felt peace within his soul. Like their owners, immune systems respond sweetly and swiftly to peace within the soul that can alter the energy of the body, bringing peace and healing to it. Whichever it was, Job's life experiences have left us the richer for the understanding of our own, which however still beg essential questions. What is the nature of memory and the consciousness that controls and can change the functioning of our bodies, minds, and souls?

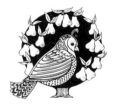

IV

The Sacred Webs of Memory

A T THE FOUNDING IN CALIFORNIA of the Mission of San Juan Capistrano in 1776, little did the Franciscan friars from Spain imagine that it would eventually become famous, not for its role in the history of California or the Spanish Empire, but for its swallows. At dawn on March 19th every year, St. Joseph's Day, the little birds begin to arrive at the Mission after having journeyed from their winter habitats in South America. Mud nests from yesteryears that still cling to the ruins of the old stone church are quickly repaired and the serious business of nesting and mating begins. Summers are spent raising their young and then on the Feast of St. Juan Capistrano, October 23, the swallows, parents and children alike, take flight to their Southern Hemisphere winter habitats. Every year the ritual of their arrival on March 19th and their departure on October 23rd is unfailingly repeated.

Spring comes late to Western New York where I live, but each year the grackles and robins, along with the doves and barn swallows arrive back from their winter abodes. Although not with the same precision as the swallows of San Juan Capistrano, nevertheless, their arrival in mid-to-late March is always a heart-warming event, heralding as it does the arrival of spring. Some take up residence under the eaves of the roof, others nest on top of the pillars as they jut out from underneath the porches they support, and others choose the barn as well as other places including the old milk shed and well house. From dawn to dusk these creatures are madly busy either repairing the vacated nests of their ancestors, some of which may have been their own birthing places and nurseries, or, as the severity of our winters often make necessary, building new ones. Then, like the famous swallows, they all get down to the business of mating and raising their fledglings. Some of these families offer me an opportunity to participate in their rituals for it is not uncommon for the greedy young ones to fall out of their nest when they have overreached in order to retrieve food from the beaks of their parents. These little fallen ones either get returned to the nest or, if the parents have flown away, I nurture them until they can fly away on their own life's journey, but with the memories of their beginnings safely tucked away under their wings to be replicated next year and the next and the next.

The sagas of nature's rituals are endless. The salmon in our streams — yes, we have them in Western New York — often make heroic journeys back to the place where they were spawned and where they, like their ancestors, will spend themselves spawning new life that will ensure the continuance of their kind into endless future generations. These and other wondrous happenings throughout and within creation have always intrigued and challenged humanity. Their precision and repetition, their inherent beauty and thrust to survival and reproduction, jostle with questions that beg knowledge of how it is all accomplished.

Obviously, memory, in particular some transgenerational aspects of it and other yet unnamed factors, drive these phenomena. But, then, one has to ask what it is that drives and directs memory with such power and elegance. Our lives and customs are engulfed by memory. The rituals and liturgies of religion and the rites of human passage are chosen for their significance in the lives of past generations, vehicles within which we feel, know, and even touch our connectedness as a continuum with all existence. As an entity, it has been the subject of much discourse throughout recorded history, discourse which has reached a crescendo of speculation and definition over the past quarter century; but, its precise nature continues to elude us. To enumerate the functions of memory is to state the obvious. It overlaps with our perceptions and with our ability to learn. It flows into and with our consciousness at all of its levels – thus, providing the stage if not also the choreography for the unfolding drama of our lives. The ancient Greeks knew this. They regarded their goddess Mnemosyne as the fount of memory and the mother of the muses. They believed that poetry, song, and drama, indeed, every creative art form, sprang from memory and would forever be rooted in it. Moreover, they believed that *memory* was the "all" of life and that, therefore, all creation was her offspring; but from where, beyond Mnemosyne, did memory arise?

Aeschylus, the great Greek philosopher, asserted that memory was the mother of all wisdom. However, in the Judaic scriptures of his time, wisdom is referred to as "she" who was before all creation. If so, then who and what is memory if she is the mother of wisdom and progenitor and transmitter of life? Pursuing her identity was for millennia the purview of philosophers and poets, a pursuit she artfully eluded with only the barest of holes in her veils. During the latter half of the 20th century scientists joined the pursuit, but put an emphasis on finding a precise location wherein she dwells. One has to wonder at the logic behind this, not only because memory is so pervasive in our lives but, because findings from sociological research makes it clear that describing location defines its inhabitants in only the most general of terms. This approach, however, is in tune with the thrust of most Western science which tends to describe phenomena by the variables associated with them, as well as in terms of their secondary characteristics of form and function rather than of their essence. Scientific sleuthing after memory has proceeded along two pathways and their attendant parameters. On the one hand, neurobiologists who assume that memory is solely a function of the brain have tried to establish its hardware by tracking the nerve cells and their neurons involved to some degree with one or an other of its numerous functions. On the other hand, psychologists have been probing the software of memory by attempting to describe its many facets and functions. One of their most important conclusions was arrived at by studying patients with varying degrees and modes of loss of memory, collectively referred to as amnesia. From this, they concluded that there is no single entity that can be called "memory." How correct they are can be confirmed by a few moments reflection on whom we are and how we came to be. For example, in all species when an egg is fertilized, and providing it escapes threats to its development, it will eventually be born as a replica of its parent(s). At the time of fertilization, there is no brain and, therefore, no road map of nerve cells and neurons to enable its inherent memory of who it is to proceed through the growth and development that culminates in it replicating its progenitors. In fact, so certain are we that this elusive entity, called memory, will reproduce its own kind, we rarely give it a thought in the begetting of our own children. Likewise, when mice and other mammalians are bred in research laboratories, it never occurs to us that a mouse might produce an elephant or that an elephant and other species in the wild would reproduce anything other than their own kind. Surely, then, it is obvious that memory by any other name is not only within and at the very heart and center of creation, but goes before it in all of its manifestations. Memory is primal to our existence.

Furthermore, recent advances in neurophysiology have delineated some of the orderly electrochemical and energy bases of how we function. That these are transmitted trans-generationally confirms what perennial wisdom has always known — all life and its sustaining functions are encoded in memory and, therefore, memory is everywhere within the body and soul — not just in one place. We come into life because of memory and its legions of specificities for each and every trait of whom we are and may become, contained within our genes. A half century ago Albert Einstein told us that ultimate reality lay within fields of energy and not within particles, no matter how small. Thus, while we still conceive of genes as particulate matter which, indeed, they are, we know the driving force behind their activities must be energy. We know, too, that all functions of our mind, body, and soul are affected through these fields of electrochemical magnetic energy which, indeed, form the bases for many medical diagnostic tests. But, since all life is encoded in memory, then memory is also energy. We also know that energy fields are acutely sensitive to all that disturbs or threatens their particular wave patterns and frequencies. When this happens, it changes the nature of their functions to the point of their dysfunction.[1] Indeed, memory operates within our beings in a manner akin to how the physical immune system functions. As already described in the previous chapter, the cells of the immune system, the substances they produce, and their receptors are thinking entities whose function is to defend against all that is *non-self* through a system of locks and keys that for the most part operates with exquisite precision and protectiveness. Sadly, there are times when the immune system dysfunctions. In some cases, it overreacts to external stimuli, e.g., in allergies and autoimmune diseases, and in oth-

---

[1]Ursula M. Anderson, *The Sacredness of Memory: Immunology and the Soul.* **Anima** (Buffalo Diocesan Liturgical Commission: Buffalo, NY), (XVII, No. 2, 1993): 13-14 (11-19 —The full article may be obtained by contacting She-Bear Publications, P. O. Box 503, Ellicottville, NY 14731).

ers, it fails to react or it underreacts. In all cases, the memory sequences of how to protect the body temple have been injured, and the precise sensitivity of that energy damaged to where it no longer can function as it was intended. The confusion and anger at this betrayal of self and self-identity is manifested by disease and disorder.

Wondrous as is all of this, how did it all get started? Eschewing for a moment the mythology that surrounds Judeo-Christian biblical accounts of Creation, scientists tell us that at the beginning there was a horrendous collision of forces in the universe that liberated atoms of carbon, hydrogen, nitrogen, and oxygen — a happening that now is referred to as the "Big Bang." Over time, these elements engaged each other in the primal dance of creation. From their various unions emerged several variations of the arrangements they made for coexistence, no doubt in each instance getting it right after much trial and error. The molecules so formed continued to dance in ever-escalating complexity to form the building blocks that over millennia became the infrastructure and basis of plant life and unicellular organisms – all eventually evolving into the human form.

At every step of the way, it can be assumed that constant adjustments had to be made not only to permit the wondrous diversity and healthy unfolding of species-specific life, but also to allow for responses to the environments within which they were made. It is a dialogue that continues to this day, but within which environment is presently taking on the more talkative and dominant role — and not always a beneficial one. Pitting this negative trend against the majesty of creation, one prays and works for it to be halted and stopped in its tracks. Glimmers of the majesty of creation are evident throughout recorded history and in this century described in compelling and deeply spiritual terms by the great paleontologist and priest Pierre Teilhard de Chardin. Several decades of paleontological research, carried out mostly in China (and what a lonely task that must have been only he knew), led him to conceive of creation as an unfolding of the human spirit through time and the destination of its journey a return to its source in God. Despite the call of history to the contrary, de Chardin also believed that this journey was never without memories of its beginnings.[2] This point of resonance with the thinking of Carl Jung, who believed that humankind carries memories of the past in its collective consciousness, brings to mind yet again the coherence of thought in the evolution of human consciousness.

More recently, in writing about the power of memory and energy and their many manifestations, Rupert Sheldrake suggested that there is an energy that holds the blueprints for species-specific morphology and function whose duties may be compared to that of a monitor that he calls "Morphic Resonance."[3] It has also been described as an entity that somehow, by establishing habits, prompts other memories what to do. If this is so, then, juxtaposing it with electrochemical and other energies inherent in genes, it seems reasonable to deduce that if, following conception, they are out of tune with each other during early development, attempts will be made to correct this dissonance in the interest of preserving morphological and functional integrity and purity. That such is, in fact, the case is strongly supported by a unique epidemiological study conducted on the island of Kauai in Hawaii over a period of 20 years commencing in 1955.[4]

Beginning in the prenatal period, the Kauai study followed all the children who survived in an entire community representing all

---

[2]Pierre Teilhard de Chardin, *Human Energy* (New York, NY: Harcourt Brace) English Translation (London,UK: William Collins, 1969).

[3]Rupert Sheldrake, *A New Science of Life*. (Cambridge, UK: Cambridge University Press, 1981); and *The Presence of the Past*. (Cambridge, UK: Cambridge University Press, 1988).

[4]Werner, Bierman and French, *The Children of Kauai*, 1971: Werner and R. Smith, *Kauai's Children Come of Age*, (Hawaii: University of Hawaii Press), 1977.

socioeconomic and ethnic groups on the island and maintained the cooperation of 90% of them throughout the second decade of life. The study addressed many parameters of child development and the consequences of the threats and stresses that occurred in the perinatal period defined as from 20 weeks of gestation to 28 days of life. Overall, the researchers provided a wealth of information that seems not to have received the attention it deserves. However, regarding its relation to this polemic, it was reported that of pregnancies reaching 4 week's gestation, an estimated 237 per 1000 ended in loss of the conceptus. The rate of loss formed a decreasing curve from as high as 108/1000 women under observation in the period of 4 to 7 weeks of gestation to a low of 3/1000 in the period of 32 to 35 weeks of gestation. What this indicates is that when, for whatever reason or reasons, genetic memories and energies are damaged in the process of being passed from one generation to another, and therefore cannot jibe, respond, or interact with others and the protective memory of morphic resonance, there are consequences. These range along a linear path of those so severe, resulting in death to the conceptus, which, from this data, would appear to happen in a surprisingly high proportion of pregnancies, to the least severe, allowing intrauterine development to continue to birth but with some injury to morphology and/or function at some stage or even throughout independent life.

The Kauai study sheds light on these outcomes. The perinatal mortality rate, based on fetal deaths of 20 weeks or more and on infant deaths under 28 days, was 35.9% per 1000 pregnancies. Of the remaining live-born infants, by age two 3.7% were diagnosed as severely handicapped, requiring long-term medical or custodial care, while 6.3% were diagnosed with conditions requiring short-term medical or nursing care. However, by age 10, 6.6% of the children were deemed moderately or severely handicapped as a result of physical or mental defects or both. Of these, over five times as many children required special *educational* services (39%) as those who required *medical* care and almost twice as many had emotional and behavioral problems interfering with school progress (13%).

In summation, for an estimated 1311 pregnancies that had advanced to 4 week's gestation, 10 years later only 660 children, that is, half the pregnancies, were functioning adequately in school and had no "recognized" physical, intellectual, or behavioral problems. While it should be noted that depending on the severity of the dysmorphism and dysfunction resulting from dissonance in genetic and other memories — the most severe of these conditions themselves interrupt their replication by rendering their victims infertile — this study and others clearly point to other very important and fundamental issues. First, memory — whatever its nature and residence – reaches not only for physical survival but also, more importantly, for physical integrity. The high degree of casualties following fertilization reflects nature's bent to perfection, not so much by not making mistakes but, once made, by seeking to remedy them. This is a theme, if not also a deep knowing, echoed by Henry Skolimowski's imagery in his book *"The Theater of the Mind,"* in which he says, "Glory to evolution, for it is God. God is evolution realizing itself: transforming us into more and more radiant fragments of Godliness. We are God in the making. We learn the meaning of God in the process of becoming one. The terror of this realization must not be license for arrogance but an invitation to humility."

Second, and closely related to the first, while there have been a few exemplary studies pointing to the fact that emotional and behavioral problems in children and adults manifest early in life, the Kauai study clearly documents the early genesis and long-term fallout of injured memories that have their impact on the expression of the soul. The coherence between damage to the memories that affect the physical body and those that affect the soul and the mind is that, evidently, they both occur very early in development. In recent years much has been written about soul, all of which has been enriching for where we are in our journeyings. Yet, the origins of soul still beg enlightenment, as does, also, its very nature.

The mere utterance of "soul" creates rivers of feelings and memories within our being. Indeed, we frequently evoke and invoke soul to convey depths of feelings that defy description in words, as the word itself invites and then teasingly defies precise definition. The Oxford Universal Dictionary devotes almost an entire page in attempting to describe it. As with consciousness, our Western approach to defining substance by listing its attributes is evident. Soul is described among other things as the seat of feelings and emotion — the feeling and spiritual part of our human nature and the Principle of Life. But, the source of all life is God, and all life is encoded in memory. Therefore, soul can be perceived as that which is eternal, containing the memory of our beginnings in God and which, throughout our lives, seeks living union with its source. Furthermore, if we take its characteristics as reflective of its essence, it is the feeling part of us that connects us to the Sacred of our origins; and, since we share our origins with all of creation, it is also that which connects us with each other. Soul is therefore, among other things but, primarily, that which gives us a sense of our own unique identity and, within the quality of its early memories, our capacity or otherwise to relate to others. If these memories are injured, we will suffer in varying degrees from a diminution or loss of self-identity and the ability to relate soulfully to others.

Over the past century or so, certainly since the time of Freud, disturbances of self-identity and relatedness have been perceived as disorders of thought around which have developed countless theories and therapies of psychology and psychiatry. Perhaps we miss the meaning of psychology and psychiatry for the root of both words derives from *Psyche* who was the God of the Soul. While it is inevitable that disorders of self-identity and inter-personal relatedness result in disorders of thought, perception, feelings and behavior, the disorders themselves have their origins in memories. We now know that the texture of our feelings and, thus, our behavioral tendencies are woven from the fabric of our early sensory and emotional experience beginning, many scientists believe, in the prenatal period, if not before.

While these early experiences are beyond our conscious recall, the memories of them, modified by the memories of feelings passed to us in our genes from our parents and their forebears, become the initial locks and keys of how we will "feelingly" respond to life. In other words, our initial encounters form the bases upon which all other experience will be grafted and interpreted. Likewise, it sets the stage for how immune our soul will be to the experiences of life that seek to disconnect us from our true heritage as children of God and of Love. If these initial encounters are loving and welcoming, they will create positive, nurturing memories in the soul, thus creating strong immunization against the effects of all that subsequently seeks to disconnect it from its source and facilitating our ability to relate positively to others. If these encounters are not loving or welcoming, the memories so created provide weak immunization against the assaults that seek to separate the soul from the source of its life in God, thus, diminishing our ability to relate with others. If not ameliorated by therapy and/or other means and, indeed, if reinforced by later experience, these negative memories lead to feelings of worthlessness, hopelessness, and ultimately to a belief that all that is external to oneself is hostile. Surely, the small step from this to overt violence is clearly evident. How all of this plays out in our later life becomes a drama of cosmic proportions.

Allow me to introduce the drama by describing in scientific terms the likely long-term effects of our initial sensory encounters. Recent research has found that if a newborn infant is not held skin-to-skin with its mother within six hours of birth, the chemistry of neurotransmission in the amygdala nucleus located in the limbic system — which is that part of the brain that controls emotion and feeling — changes. The amygdala nucleus modulates levels of aggression through its role as coordinator of sensory input from the neo-cortex. This results in the activation of the hypothalamus which is the part of the brain that controls the autonomic system and, likewise, has direct and controlling connections to the endocrine system, as well as the immune system. Here is where the experiential drama begins. The autonomic nervous system controls every function of the body and is the reason why the energy of feelings is felt throughout the body. Thus, from shortly after birth, our later tendencies to aggressivity or passivity that are derived from feelings, as well as our gut reactions to threat – whether real or perceived – are stamped in the memory banks of our soul. These feelings cast a shadow over or enhance the primal memory of our beginnings in God. This is why it is so essential that infants cared for in neonatal intensive care units be touched, held, and stroked in a loving, reassuring way as often as possible.[5] The intention is to counteract the long-term effects of the somewhat violent nature of the invasive needle and other procedures necessary to save their lives which create memories of violent feelings that could then influence later experience. Without this intervention, these infants may become candidates for Reactive Attachment Disorder of Infants and Early Childhood (RADIEC) which results from poor or absent bonding at birth and manifests as emotional and behavioral dysfunction throughout childhood and later life. In addition, other recent observations on emotional development in children indicate that the constancy of loving and nurturing contact with the mother in the first six months of life facilitates the subsequent ability to make and maintain healthy human relationships. Does all this point to the validation of the old axiom, "The hand that rocks the cradle, rules the world?" It certainly seems so and, as such, has a profound message if we have the ears to hear in terms of redressing the soul sickness and violence in our society that has reached epidemic proportion.

Recent data from the *U.S. Longitudinal Study on Children and*

[5] *Journal of Pediatrics* (January 1993).

Adolescence suggests that 29% of children between the ages of seven and fourteen have severe emotional, behavioral, and learning disorders — not just any disorder, but a severe disorder. Since fear and anxiety result from negative experiences and are inherent components of these disorders, it behooves us to make the connection and to facilitate and encourage mothers, by whatever means, to lovingly nurture their infants and children. Since many themselves come to motherhood deprived of positive nurturing, the task is formidable, but not impossible. Indeed, as more and more of the secrets of God's creation unfold, motherhood is revealed as the most sacred of vocations and occupations bar none. Indeed, if the sacredness of mothering was promoted and fostered, I venture to say that if all other factors were equal the proclivity to violence would be substantially diminished.

Important as these experiences immediately following birth may be, they are preceded by what happens from conception throughout prenatal life. But there is more. Many people today are aware of the deleterious and often catastrophic effects on the fetus and newborn child due to the mother's drug use during pregnancy. Some of these effects include premature birth — along with all of the hazards associated with it, including growth retardation, microcephaly, birth defects, and other conditions that seriously jeopardize the quality of life for the child — which, of course, has its fallout on all of society. In some jurisdictions throughout the world, drug-using mothers-to-be have been sent to jail for endangering the lives of their infants. When separated from their mothers, this only inflicts more injury on the child. However, what is even less well known is how the thoughts, feelings, and moods of the mother impact upon the unborn child. In his book *The Secret World of the Unborn Child*, Thomas Verney vividly describes these reactions, all of which become imprinted in their memory banks.[6] Leaning on the con-

---

[6]Thomas Verney, *The Secret Life of the Unborn Child* (New York, NY: Delta Publishing, 1987).

cepts of holography — that the memory of the whole is in even the tiniest part of the whole — Stanislaus Grof, in his book *The Holotropic Mind*, goes a step further.[7] He codified the memories of conception and of intrauterine, as well as perinatal experience into what he terms four Basic Perinatal Matrices, or BPMs. Perinatal is defined, in this context, as the time interval between conception and the twenty-eighth day of postnatal life.

The first matrix, BPM-1, which can be called the "amniotic universe," refers to our experiences in the womb prior to the onset of delivery. This means that what happens to the mother in terms of her thoughts, feelings, and behavior becomes memories within the soul of the yet unborn child.

The second matrix, BPM-2, refers to cosmic engulfment with no exit. It pertains to our experiences when uterine contractions begin but before the cervix opens to liberate us.

The third matrix, BPM-3, refers to the death and rebirth struggles of our lives, and reflects our experiences of moving through the birth canal.

The fourth matrix, BPM-4, is the death and rebirth theme that is related to our experiences when we leave the mother's body.

Dr. Grof claims that each perinatal matrix has its own specific biological, psychological, and spiritual aspects and that they not only incorporate the Archetypes of Jung, but are the memories from which we react to the circumstances of our human journey. Though his theories are fascinating, and from my clinical work I believe have validity, nevertheless, his greatest contribution has been in the quest for rebirthing — by way of holotropic breathing — for those souls who, because of traumatic memories have profound and dysfunctional emotional and behavioral disorders. In this endeavor, Grof

_____

[7]Stanislaus Grof, *The Holotropic Mind* (San Francisco, CA: HarperCollins, 1990).

attempted, as did the great psychologist Abraham Maslow, to de-pathologize the human psyche and to look at the inner core of our being — the spiritual core described by Viktor Frankl[8] — not only as the source of metaphysical darkness and illness, but as the source of health and the well-spring of human creativity, the heart of how we change the milieu within which we live. Enabling children to accomplish this can literally change their lives and how they perceive themselves.

In my work with children, while breathing quietly during relaxation, they will often, and quite spontaneously, be in touch with the memories of their conception and intrauterine life from which we can enter into healing of negative experiences that were associated with it. The power of these memories is further supported by research about newborn behavior. This indicates that memory supports all their cognitive activity such as learning and communication — making their abilities in this regard appear to be innate, i.e., having arrived with them rather than resulting from a progression of development. Making use of such innate talents, newborns demonstrate both memory and intelligence as they discriminate novel from familiar stimuli and thus vigorously shape their environment to meet their needs.

These recent perspectives not only provide a context of credibility for the many signs of birth memory and consequences of birth trauma that have emerged repetitively and have been reported on over the past 100 years or so, but they relegate to history many traditional beliefs about the brain. Included among these is the idea that early parts of the brain lie idle until more important parts are developed which is reminiscent of John Locke's dictum that infants wait upon their elders to fill their minds. Likewise, it strongly suggests that the conduction of impulses, electrochemical or otherwise, along nerve fibers is certainly not the sole or major means of com-

[8]Victor Frankl, *Man's Search for Meaning* (Boston, MA: Beacon Press, 1963).

munication in the nervous system. In fact, memory — and it must be transgenerational memory — is at work from the moment of conception — and even before — to equip them to be thinking, feeling and responsive individuals ready to dialogue and even change for the better the adult world — if it were only wise enough to dialogue with them. Herein, of course, lies the great hope for immunizing the soul. While early memories are the last to leave us, we yet hold to notions that childhood memories become buried under the weight of experience — even in small children. However, one study found that two and a half year-olds remembered events that happened 9 to 12 months previously — suggesting and confirming that early memories stay in the mind and, therefore, can be accessed.[9]

Indeed, evidence for the forever-ness of holotropic memory received a spectacular endorsement as a result of the cloning of Dolly, the ewe, in 1997. Once the memories of how to behave as a cell in the mammary gland of the donor ewe were shut off, the genetic blueprints of memories for making the entire animal were set free. Interestingly, this cell had to be implanted into an egg cell from another sheep from which the nucleus had been removed because only the egg cell contains the proteins, and their attendant energies, necessary to turn on the genes and to keep them on their developmental track. Two years after the fact, Dolly is showing signs that she is genetically older than her chronological age; in fact, about the same age as the ewe from which she was cloned, which all goes to show how pervasive is genetic memory and its energy.

Further evidence for the eternity and power of holotropic memory is to be found in the behavior of microorganisms. Successful as immunization against many diseases has been, we have to be on guard against their re-emergence. Immunization is, as has already

---

[9]David B. Chamberlain in "Outer Limits of Memory," *Noetic Sciences Review,* Autumn, 1990.

been described, protection against the consequences of infection. It is not protection against invasion by infective organisms. A lead article highlighted this in the October 1995 issue of Vaccine Bulletin, which warned against a possible epidemic of diphtheria in the West, a disease most physicians presently in practice in the Western world have never seen. This concern arose because of the possibility that the diphtheria organism could be imported from the now independent states of the former Soviet Union where epidemics were occurring at that time. These were thought to derive from troops returning from Afganistan to the suboptimal levels of herd immunity in their home communities. A similar scenario is occurring with tuberculosis. In this instance, however, it would seem to derive from a natural ebb and flow to the power of infectivity of the causative organism, *Mycobacterium tuberculi*. After a steady decline from 53.0/100,000 in 1953 to 9.3/100,000 in 1985, it began to rise and is now emerging as a potentially serious health problem. Similar patterns have occurred in the past with other organisms, notably the streptococcus and its family of many cousins, particularly *beta streptococcous-group A*, that are responsible for scarlet fever, rheumatic fever, and other conditions. Thus, though the memories are always there, something interjects to change the degree of their expression. One assumes that this must be due to changes in the balance of energies within the organisms, their hosts and potential victims, and the environment within which they meet and respond to each other.

Though there is endless more to tell about memory, nevertheless, I think it is necessary to briefly mention the controversies presently engulfing what is referred to as "Repressed Memory." It has become a major problem for counselors evrywhere and has caused great suffering. Responsible counseling demands that clients should essentially be in control of their own journey into healing, with the reassuring and measured guidance of a professional, proficient counselor — much like, but different in its non-directiveness from, the free association that is used in psychoanalysis. Since all counseling is a dialogue of sorts between counselor and the one being counseled, repressed memories can emerge in two major ways. First, the client seeks counseling because of dysfunctional feelings and behavior that are making their lives painful, if not intolerable. Memories of feelings of rejection experienced from the moment of birth, during infancy and childhood that are interfering with their lives can, I believe, by an internal process of transference during counseling, be channeled into avenues of recall of physical and/or sexual abuse which may or may not have happened. A climate such as is active presently, wherein abuse of all kinds has high visibility, may serve to heighten the possibility of this happening. Nevertheless, it should be borne in mind that the emotional pain and consequences of rejection, which is abuse in and of itself, can be just as serious as those resulting from physical or sexual abuse. Of course, memories of actual physical and sexual abuse can also be suppressed. Second, a counselor may inadvertently give suggestions to a client as to what may have happened in their past. These may become imprinted in the client's recall as actual happenings in their lives which, due to their painful overtones, have been repressed in their waking consciousness. The effects of these so-called repressed memories are then perceived as the cause of the client's present dysfunction and disability. Since uncovering the cause of suffering is relief in itself, it is easy to see how these "enabled memories" become the focus of the client's pursuit of resolution. In my opinion, until we have a clearer vision of the dynamic inherent in repressed memory and its phenomena, we should not deny its existence as a powerful progenitor of human dysfunction and suffering. However, we should be very cautious about using it at face value in an accusatory way that affects the lives and well being of people the counselee may identify as their persecutors. Until such time, we should call this phenomenon, Enabled Memories.

From all of the foregoing it is clear that memory is an exquisite tapestry of many colorful threads; some of which we share with all of humanity, some which are personal to us. Carl Jung referred to those that are a shared inheritance as the *Collective Unconscious*, and described them in terms of archetypes. These interact with our own prenatal and perinatal memories, as well as those of our early childhood to become the matrix of the consciousness that drives us in body, mind, and soul and the personalities we thereby become. In seeking the causes of our *felt* sense of separation from source, which injures our own sense of personal identity — as well as our ability to relate to others — we need to look to the quality of memories in our soul. Their profundity is reflected in the story of one American couple's noble attempt to give love to an abused child from Russia. In *"Love Isn't always Enough,"* their anguish is described in the following letter to the editor that appeared in the July 7, 1997 issue of *Newsweek*.

Love Isn't Always Enough

My husband and I adopted a 10-year-old girl from Russia with no preparation for the horror to come ("Bringing Kids All the Way Home," LIFESTYLES, June 16). She came from a severely alcoholic family in which she had to steal food to survive. Her father knifed her, her mother was a prostitute and her brother sexually molested her. She lived on the street for a year before going into the orphanage at the age of 9. I received none of this information until she began speaking English and told me herself. The year my daughter lived with us was hell. She was like a wild animal in our home. Eventually, she was diagnosed as being severely disturbed with attachment disorder and aggressive tendencies. We were warned to put alarms on her bedroom door to protect ourselves from her at night. We couldn't live like this. In the most heartbreaking decision I've ever made, we disrupted our adoption. I feel very strongly that agencies need to obtain the same in-depth infor-

mation about both prospective adoptive children and prospective adoptive parents. To bring a severely disturbed child into an unprepared family sets both the child and the parents up for failure.

Another letter of equal importance followed this report. This second letter positioned for review the precise dilemma at hand.

*I was disappointed at the softness of **Newsweek's** piece on international adoption. Contrary to Bethany DeNardo's assertion, saying that with 'stimulation and loving care and good food' the kids can 'bounce back' is terribly unfair to both adoptive parents and their children. With your research and access to so many scientific studies and facts, you could have enabled readers to begin to understand some of the horrific problems associated with some adoptions of post-institutionalized children. I realize that this tough issue is not easy to look at, but it is an important story that needs to be told.*

Not until we penetrate and change the negative energies of such powerful, hurtful, and destructive memories will we ever be able to create the positive energies that will nurture and enrich a functional consciousness of self and *other*.

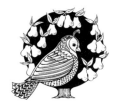

V

Original Sin, Original Identity, and The Journey of Human Consciousness

T HE BOOK OF GENESIS is the first book of the Hebrew scriptures which, nowadays, is most frequently referred to as the Old Testament of the Judeo-Christian scriptures. It tells the story of Creation and that on the sixth day God declared, "Let us make man in our image and after our likeness."[1] God did and was well pleased. So well pleased was God, in fact, that on the seventh day

---

[1]Genesis 1: 26a (New American Bible edition).

God rested from the labor of creation. Soon thereafter, feeling refreshed and renewed, God took a trip to the Garden of Eden. Herein dwelt all the plants and birds and animals that God had created before He made man and over which He now gave him dominion.

This man apparently wanted for nothing, including the personal attention of God. It was Paradise! However, did he know it? Evidently, not, for when God encountered the man, much to his surprise He found him unhappy. On questioning him, the man confided that he was lonely. "Hmm," said God, "let me think about this and see what I can do to rectify it." A few days later God visited the man again. Observing that he looked rather tired, God suggested that the man take a nap, which he did. When God saw the energy waves of Stage 4 of the sleep cycle emanating from the man's head, He performed the quickest transplant in all of medical history. Swiftly opening the man's chest through the smallest of incisions, God removed the twelfth rib on the man's right side — the smallest of all he possessed. Then, showering divine energy on it, within an instant God created a companion for the man, now called Adam, and He called this creation, Woman — SHE who would shortly thereafter become the means whereby all the furies of Hell were said to have been let loose.

Not too long after her debut in the Garden of Eden, Eve, as the woman was now called, began to feel lonesome herself and thought that there must be more to life than just being a companion to Adam. One day, perceiving her discontent, a snake engaged Eve in conversation.

"There is more than this to life you know," the snake said. "You were made for greater things than just being with man."

"Oh, really?" asked Eve. "Tell me more."

"Well," said the snake, "all you have to do is eat the fruit of the

Tree of Knowledge and you will become like God, knowing good and evil."

"How can that be?" replied Eve. Do you not know that despite this story of me being just a rib, I am Wisdom, and was before all creation? And besides, God told us not to eat of the fruit of that tree."

"Well, Knowledge is different from Wisdom," replied the snake. "But, putting that aside, don't you think that since you were an afterthought in God's plan for Creation, you should attempt to equalize that by gaining knowledge as well as wisdom? Believe me, if you eat the fruit of that tree, you can gain everlasting fame."

"How so?" asked Eve.

"Well, the story will be told that, because of your disobedience, you are to blame for all the evil that befalls mankind and this will rest on you for evermore."

"Oh!" said Eve. "I'm not sure I believe you but, then, maybe that would be better than being bored. I'll take the fruit!"

Crunching into the apple, she said, "This is delicious! I must share it with Adam." And so, she did. He accepted it willingly and agreed with Eve that it tasted good.

When God learned of what had happened, He made a hasty trip back to the Garden. Hearing Him moving about, Adam and Eve hid themselves in the bushes.

"Where are you?" God called out.

"I am hiding," replied Adam.

"Come here before me," commanded God. Adam did as he was told.

"Why are you hiding? What have you done?" demanded God. "Did I not forbid to you to eat of the fruit of the Tree of Knowledge?"

"I believe so," replied Adam.

"Yes or no?" demanded God.

"Hmm. Yes, but Eve made me do it!"

Looking sad, as well as stern, God told Adam to bring the woman to Him because what He had to say applied to both of them. Whereupon, Adam told the woman to leave her hiding place and stand with him before God. Without asking her if what Adam had said was true, God pronounced to them both that, due to their disobedience, they could no longer live in Paradise and that they both must leave the Garden immediately. Furthermore, from henceforward, Woman and her descendents would be associated with the serpent of deception, thereby subject forevermore to Man, who would be the arbiter of the essence, the quality, and the boundaries of her life.

Shortly after being banished from Paradise, and presumably because their new-found knowledge informed them of the possibilities inherent in their nakedness, a condition they previously had not noticed, they begat two sons, Cain and Abel, who became famous as the progenitors of the destructive energies inherent in sibling rivalry. Engendered by resentment, jealousy and its resulting blind hatred, Cain murdered his brother Abel — not because of any personal hurt inflicted upon his person, nor of any other wrongdoing, but, simply because Cain perceived Abel to be God's favorite.

Following the death of Abel, Adam and Eve, the primal parents of Genesis, were left with one son and no daughters — or at least none that we have been told about. Yet, the biblical narrative continues by recounting the names and activities of countless generations that followed. The gullibility that would accept such an improbable story really tests the limits of imagination. Indeed, as a story of creation, Genesis has long been submerged under the weight of paleontological and other scientific research, evidence which reveals Creation to have been a phenomenon of incredible majesty evolving over several thousands of millennia. But, as a mythic tale of how evil and suffering entered the human domain, as well as how it has remained there pursuing its own trajectory of evolution, it is a masterful backdrop to the human condition.

In pre-Genesis Hebrew culture, the presence of God, the Shekhinah, was referred to in the feminine. In fact, there were a number of gods (Elohim), both male and female, bearing many names. Lilith was "She" who was the creator of life and who, herself, had emerged from the great Mother Earth, the begetter of all natural and human life and of all religions — who was and who is both matrix and nurturer. Yet, the rabbinical writers of Genesis chose to ignore Lilith and replaced her with Eve whom they portrayed as the destroyer of life in its wholesome, creative holiness and oneness with all creation. By excluding Lilith from the picture, they conspired to masculinize God in toto and then promoted Him as the great creator. This led to a belief in the superiority of the male and the inferior status of the female, as well as her offspring, which latter permits the use and abuse of women and children. This trespass on the original sacred identity of women and children is at the center of the continuing confusion about the roles expected of men, women and children and the destructive behaviors and misery that flow from it.

That such a dramatic change in values and beliefs, and their subsequent long-term residence in the collective consciousness of humankind, could be accomplished by a few (rabbinical) writers is testimony to the power of the written and spoken word. Their monumental betrayal and subversion of what had previously been believed begs the question — why? Why did they do this? As in all such similar human situations, fear of what was being betrayed, accompanied by lust for power and control, was undoubtedly fuel to its fire. In this instance, what was being betrayed was the power of the creative and spiritual *feminine* which, alas, is still very evident today as it has been throughout the post Genesis, Judaic, and Christian eras and perhaps deriving from a memory echoing in the male consciousness of the maleness that wrought the change. How it was done is another mystery — maybe a slip of the pen or, as some scholars suggest, a poor choice in subsequent interpretation. The fact that the text would and can bear constructs equally acceptable scholastically, but which would change its message and meaning, suggests the use of deliberate license with interpretation. Then, of course, it could have been a well-thought-out way of transferring feminine power to the masculine experience, but, over all the theories rests the certainty that barring divine intervention, we shall never know the real reason(s) of *why* and *how*. Nevertheless, what took place changed the way much of how humankind had previously perceived itself — which was as people of the land, forest, and sea, intimately related to the Earth, as Mother, and living as an egalitarian, *shamanic* society whose spirituality was centered on unity and immanence — the *Shekhinah*. By so doing, it undeniably fractured its *wholeness*.

Commenting on this perfidy, Judith Plaskow observed that a god who does not include the goddess is an idol made in man's image.[2] Theologian Elizabeth Schussler-Fiorenza cautions that androcentric texts and linguistic constructions must *not* be mistaken as trustworthy evidence of human culture and religion.[3] This thought is echoed by Bernadette Brooten who has surveyed Jewish

---

[2]Judith Plaskow, "The Right Question Is Theological" in *On Being A Jewish Feminist*, S. Heschel (Ed.). (Schocken: New York, 1983).

[3]Elisabeth Schussler-Fiorenza, *In Memory of Her*. (Crossroads: New York, 1983). Reading of her other works is highly recommended by this author.

and Hellenistic inscriptions and suggests that literature composed by men is the product of men's minds and not a simple mirror image of reality.[4] These latter two are strong statements and while one could enter a polemic regarding the nature of reality, nevertheless, within a historical perspective they are probably fair comment.

Adding to the mystery of why Genesis was written is its timing. Understandably, there is uncertainty about the dates of the writing and compilation of the Hebrew bible. Some scripture scholars place the writing of Genesis after the period of the compilation of the Law and the Prophets, which took place approximately in the early 400s BCE (Before the Common Era). Yet, the events the bible describes took place centuries earlier — 1800 BCE for the time of Abraham and from about 900 BCE for David and Solomon. This raises the possibility that Genesis, or parts of it, were afterthoughts, albeit in hindsight afterthoughts with an agenda whose program of reconditioning and refocusing mind, soul, and behavior is still very much with us.

Further intrigue is added when, as a chronicle of Creation, it is compared with the Creation stories and myths of other religions. In general, it may be said these conceive Creation to be emanations from God who is more often than not regarded as being both male and female. These emanations, which I surmise are currents of eternal energy, initially entered and subsequently re-enter into eternal cycles of integration, disintegration, and reintegration. There are many cultural variations on this theme, of which in its own way Genesis is one. It addresses integration as the experience of Adam and Eve in the Garden of Eden and disintegration as their expulsion from it following their so-called disobedience. For the Jewish people, reintegration awaits the arrival of a Messiah who, it is believed,

---

[4]Bernadette Brooten, *Women Leaders in the Ancient Synagogue.* (Scholars Press: California, 1982).

will end their exodus and reestablish them as God's *chosen*. How *He*, and again the emphasis is on the male, will accomplish this is not clear. It is worth noting, however, that it has frequently been suggested that the salvation or reintegration that is hoped for will not come from an "other" but from within the heart and soul of each individual — much as some latter-day theologians suggest that Christ Jesus understood salvation as God's intimate involvement with human life here and now, rather than being mediated by another or hierarchies who have assumed ownership and control over it and its fruits.

Christianity refers to the Hebrew bible as the Old Testament and subscribes to its contents as being the forerunner of the New Testament which chronicles the life of Jesus, the Christ, whom Christians accept as the much hoped for Messiah. He it is, who through his life and death, redeems or reintegrates the consequences of the fall from God's grace of Adam and Eve. This is an event conceptualized and referred to as the *Original Sin*, whose imprint is said to be on every human being and which in Christianity is said to be washed away by baptism. Original sin as a concept, *per se*, is unique to Christianity and it is often referred to as the sin of our first parents. However, if there were no first parents called Adam and Eve, where does this leave original sin? As a singular event in time and space, it is almost certainly a nonhappening. Yet, its hold on the human imagination remains and not without reason because it is intimately related to original identity and, indeed, is perceived as the reason original identity was lost.

As a religious text, Genesis became doctrine, and doctrine is that which must be believed. It is a doctrine that set the stage and thereafter provided the *imprimatur* for the superiority and dominance of men — from which they assumed authority and control over women and children. Women and children were thereby effectively expelled to the nether regions of subjugation and servitude. Thus was stolen their sacred original identity as the vessels of creation and fecundity and the seeds of forever future generations.

This was and this remains the Original sin!

It was the sword with which humankind wounded and still wounds itself — a wound that lies open and weeping, awaiting its healing. Alas, it is not the only wound of which Genesis speaks and which, if we match it with human experience through the ages, leads us into an understanding of the consequences of the loss of our original identity. The story tells us that in the Garden of Eden, there was direct contact with God and the consciousness of man and woman was in tune with the consciousness of all creation. It was perfect; it was integration; it *was* paradise. There was immunity from all that could destroy it. When paradise was lost, disintegration followed. As generation followed generation, immunity to that which could injure or destroy unity with self, others, and with all creation was weakened and became vulnerable to these assaults. Thus, over time, the memories of unity and immanence grew dim, but as with all memories, they were never totally lost. These memories speak to us in the depths of our souls; they remain that still small voice that prompts us to reach and to grasp the love of its origin and which yearns for reintegration with its source. However, pursuing the story as it unfolds, it becomes clear that subsequent to the "Fall," reintegration had to be worked at, using the self-same knowledge that caused it. Fortunately, we are also blessed with intuition, perception, and other gifts which, together with knowledge, enable us to assess the environments within and external to us and to interpret what their interplay may or may not mean in relation to one's self and to others. The thoughts and feelings so generated will be a medley of the memories of integration and its loss, which if in balance is positive and will manifest as functional and, if negative, will manifest as dysfunctional behavior. Intertwined with this are the consequences of the loss of blissful naturalness that yielded to the scramble to cover nakedness, not only of body, but also of mind and soul. The resulting anxiety and inner sense of disconnectedness then become major conctituents in the matrix of the mask we present to others to cover our insecurities and which we use in the struggle for power, control, and supremacy.

Thus, over time, thoughts and feelings have entered into an intimate relationship with perceptions and interpretations that has served to further cloud the memory of integration and harmony that existed in Paradise. This, in turn, generated other memories of *how* self should respond in self-protection and preservation to all that was external and nonself. These alterations and additions served to change not only individual consciousness, but ultimately the collective consciousness as well.

While it is feasible to lay the ills of body, mind, and soul within the consequences of disintegration, yet, because our theme is soul, it is particularly appropriate to examine them within that context. In our culture, sickness of soul is often identified with sickness of mind and, of course, the two are connected if not also intertwined; but here I will use the term "psychiatric" to imply sickness of the soul with the understanding that this almost always accompanies sickness of the mind. No matter what the cause of the soul sickness or specific psychiatric diagnosis may be, and regardless of its particular manifestations and symptoms, at the core of each and all of them is the disharmony that results from a profound sense of disconnection from the harmony of source and its resulting anxiety and fear. The battlefield wherein these memories jostle each other for supremacy results in "stress." Though the word itself is now part of the vernacular, few are aware of nor do they fully understand the physiological changes that constitute the body's reaction to stress with its overflow to mind and soul — which is called the "Stress Response." Although it will be described in some detail later, suffice it here to say that during the stress response, memories and energies within body, mind, and soul that facilitate our healthful functioning are altered. The effects of these alterations can range from temporary to irrecoverable dysfunction. The more severe the dysfunction, so much dimmer the memory of original identity becomes. Choreographing this scenario with the march of millions of people throughout thousands of millennia, it becomes almost impossible to imagine the billions of changes that have occurred in the scenes that are the play of the memories of form and function of body, mind, and soul since the time of human oneness with Creation. Collectively they have been both blessing and curse, on the one hand enabling our continuance on this planet and at the same time when positive adaptation was not achieved becoming the source of our sicknesses.

We know that geography, topography, climate, altitude, and the practices of different cultures, among other factors, helped to modify the response to stress, thus creating differences in the resulting genetic alterations of form and function passed from generation to generation. However, it must be said that we are at a point in history when the negative effects of these changes as they affect human behavior are so profound that dysfunction in the form of violence at all levels of society is the norm. If we humans are a reflection, albeit a much dimmed one, of the face of God, then what in addition to the changes that have occurred over millennia is presently happening to bring about what appears to be an acceleration in its defacement? That such is happening seems not to be in question and, in fact, is the concern of people everywhere.

This universal concern was highlighted by the cover of the April 7, 1997 edition of *U.S. News and World Report*, which in bold letters spelled out, "LOST SOULS."[5] Between its covers was a cornucopia of articles addressing a variety of issues centered around negative, and self and other destructive human behaviors such as "Why People Commit Suicide; What Attracts People to Cults; How Reasonable People Hold and Adhere to What Appear to be

---

[5] *U.S. News and World Report*, "Lost Souls." (April 7, 1997).

Unreasonable Beliefs." The lead article was about trafficking in Russian women for sex businesses abroad. Perhaps the most intriguing and, in terms of human consciousness, certainly the most interesting article was "The Eternal Quest for a New Age. The Thin Line Between Faith and Zealotry, Religion and Cults."

The content and title of this article converged with all the others, inasmuch as each and all of them reflect the urge within humankind to re-connect with its creative source, the eternal call within humankind that is hungry for what is enduring. Although one may consider the methods and behaviors to be negative and self-defeating, nevertheless, these negatives themselves derive from the dimming of the memories of original identity and, in a perverse way, they may be regarded as a search for reconnection to it. A woman who eventually died in the Heavens Gate cult mass-suicide that occurred in California — at the time of the appearance of the Hale-Bopp Comet in February 1997 — in explaining why she joined the cult, put it this way: "They," i.e., the members of the Heavens Gate, "had a formula of how to get out of the human kingdom to a level above human and, I said to myself, this is what I want, this is what I have been looking for." In so saying, she gave voice to the deep hunger that gnaws within every human soul, particularly those who feel a deep inner sense of isolation and disconnectedness, to have someone else take responsibility for leading them out of their despair. No doubt, this is part of the reason why organized religions have for too long been able to promote dictates of "Do's" and "Don'ts" as conditions for membership in their churches. Such control serves only to emphasize conformity to authority, rather than the development of personal spirituality and, thus, serves to further distance the individual from "at-one-ment" with their creative source, which is what they seek. But, as if to confirm the shared heritage of humanity, all religions at their beginnings had as their central message, Love: love for the God of creation; love for oneself – not an egotistical love, but one deriving from one's source in creation — and, through this connection, love for one's neighbor, family, and, indeed, all of humankind. Love, therefore, means greeting every event and encounter as a means of showing and giving love. But, because we also share the consequences of the dimming of our original identity, we too often confront instead of encounter. Dwelling on the injuries so inflicted serves to further dim and diminish the energies inherent in love, which makes letting go of injury through forgiveness a necessary — if not essential — ingredient of it. Alas, the institutions and churches that men established ostensibly to enshrine and safeguard these messages frequently became depots for despots. Hierarchies took unto themselves worldly titles, jealously guarded the privileges they conferred on themselves, and exercised power over the rank and file by the use of fear and punishment, often unto death. Most pernicious of all was the idea they perpetrated that God could only be reached through a priestly intermediary and that a priest alone could confer reconciliation with God. The exclusion of women and children from participation in the "perks" of religion and church continues to this day. As shall be described later, the memories this has posited in the collective consciousness have played a tremendous role in human behavior to the point of how we perceive gender values and roles and the organization of society itself.

In addition to the pursuit of control over people, organized religions have been the cause of endless dissents and numerous wars, all devolving from the notion that one's own is the only "true" religion. This fosters perceptions that all others are in error and that therefore their followers are infidels to be feared or eliminated. In fact, as Elaine Pagels points out in her book *The Origin of Satan*, the early Christians shamelessly made out their opponents to be the devil.[6] The Crusades of the Middle Ages are an example of the long-term violence and bloodshed that can result from these passionately held

---

[6]Elaine Pagels, The Origin of Satan. (Random House: NY, 1995).

and, sometimes, mindless beliefs. That memories of these experiences and events dwell within the collective consciousness and play a role in collective human behavior cannot be denied. Twentieth century eruptions of ethnic, religious, and internecine wars and the unspeakable brutalities opposing sides inflict on each other confirms it. Yet, humankind yearns for this to change.

Fortunately, the messages of original identity have endured, and in no small measure due to the hidden and holy lives and activities of monks and nuns everywhere, both in the East and the West, who left us blueprints of how to be in touch with it. In this regard, it is worthy of note that while there have been Church leaders of exemplary character and holiness, relatively few saints of the Christian churches came from their hierarchies. For the most part they were souls who walked humbly with their God and came from the ranks of the ordinary. Of course, there have been others who strove for change in more visible and militant ways — all of which has made inroads into the work of touching once again our original identity. For example, although women are still not given full voice in most religions, burning them as witches or otherwise killing and maiming them because of their inherent spiritual powers, or for daring to challenge priestly or clerical authority, no longer occurs — or, at least, as far as we know. Further, rapprochement towards unity is not only occurring between sects and denominations within religions but religions themselves are in dialogue with each other. Presently, outstanding is the dialogue between Tibetan Buddhism and its leader, His Holiness the Dalai Lama, and certain elements within the world community of Christians. This was exemplified in 1994 when in London the Dalai Lama led the annual John Main Seminar — an international spiritual event held in honor and memory of Father John Main. Fr. Main was a Benedictine monk who founded the Christian Meditation Community, now a worldwide network. The title of that three-day seminar was *The Good Heart*, during the course of which the Dalai Lama rendered a Buddhist perspective on some of the teachings of Jesus Christ. The impact on the mostly Christian attendees was to say the least profound. The Dalai Lama emphasized, as he always does, that the purpose of all religions was not to build more temples, mosques, or churches out-side, but to build dwelling places of goodness and compassion inside the heart — to which, I would add "and the soul" — of every human being.

Such dialogue between religions and their leaders not only serves to create respect and reverence for differences, but at the same time, defuses fear of the other. Consequently, it promotes an awareness of the inter-connectedness of humanity within human consciousness that serves to permit the free flow of the universal and eternal messages of *love* and *forgiveness*.

Throughout history, humankind has been fascinated with con-sciousness — its nature, its power, and its role in the lives of indi-viduals, as well as within and throughout the entire human family. Like love, it is a many splendored thing. Therefore, to ask "What is consciousness?" is akin to asking "What is love?" or even "What is life itself?" In the past, it was thought to be the same as knowledge. Roger Bacon, who 700 years ago pioneered this notion, claimed that there were two ways of knowing: one by discourse and argument, and the other by experience. He believed that these two ways were complementary, neither being reducible to the other, and that the exercise of one mode simultaneously with the other was incompati-ble, if not impossible — which, of course, added yet another obsta-cle in the journey toward reintegration. The first mode, that of dis-course and argument, is rational, verbal, and sequential thus, linear and measurable. The second mode — that of experience — is intu-itive, spatial, and diffuse, thus less orderly and less susceptible to description and certainly evasive to linear description or research.

In Western culture, we have through science, education, and even religion concentrated on the first mode. Since it is linear and measurable, we have attempted to define consciousness in the objective and measurable terms of its secondary phenomena, expressed in behavior and verbalization. Thus, it is no surprise that those who have attempted to explain and describe consciousness have come predominantly from our various scientific communities. The intuitive mode of knowing — until recently largely ignored in Western culture — has been for millennia the norm of inquiry for those of Eastern cultures. This approach to knowing and consciousness places emphasis on personal, subjective, and empirical phenomena that lead to an inner awareness of *oneness* and connectedness with God and all of God's creation. Thus, it is no surprise that those who have described it, and continue to do so, come mainly from the monastic traditions of the religions into which they were born — the several paths of Buddhism, the eclecticism of Hinduism, the Tao's of Taoist Chinese philosophy, and the mystical tradition of Christianity.

The yearnings of the human soul to know and to be touched by the true meaning of its existence — which is union with God — has, in this century, evoked a search for a bridge between these polar opposite approaches to consciousness and knowing, particularly as this applies to human wholeness and holiness. The rapprochement began with religious scholars and writers from both East and West. However, in recent years it has found unlikely allies in Western neurophysiological research and the imploding field of trans-personal psychology. Both have demonstrated how, in our living and in how we live, i.e., our feelings and behavior, we are bound by the beliefs and concepts that we hold in our minds. These derive in large measure from the memories of our experience: genetic, evolutionary, and personal, as well as our conditioning and the teaching and training we have received. For example, one hundred years ago, no one in their rational (i.e., thinking) mind would have believed that by anno domini 1969 a man would land on the moon. In Western culture "moon" was unreachable, unknowable, save to poets and others who let their imaginations flow into supposedly unreal fantasy. In fact, they were, in their intuitive minds, relating to the truths of the ebb and flow of the tides of human experience often influenced — as are the tides of the seas — by the movements of the moon that create changes in the electromagnetic energy fields of the earth and within its inhabitants. Similarly, the concepts developed and subsequently taught and held within the fields of psychiatry and psychology have throughout their existence in the 20th century, in large measure, been bound by rational, self- and soul-limiting theories of human behavior. Therapy has concentrated on the personal and behavioral modalities of correction rather than on transforming the consequences of the origins of psychopathology that reside within transgenerational, genetic, and experiential memories and consciousness to which have been added the memories of personal experience. These memories become engraved on the soul and are known to the individual as thought and experienced as feelings. Since thoughts and feelings are antecedent to behavior, treating the behavioral manifestations of disordered thought and feelings without regard to cause defies logic and is akin to putting a band-aid on a skin ulcer, the cause of which is diabetes. Without treating the diabetes, the ulcer will not heal because the memory of the mechanism of its genesis is still within the body. The ulcer will continue to respond to the message of that memory until the cause is modified and so it is with all memories.

Several great minds of the 20th century have applied their skills to describing the phenomena associated with consciousness, if not also attempting to define it. The many writings of Pierre Teilhard de Chardin reveal that he conceived of consciousness as a circular journey of energy proceeding from its source, the Alpha Point, through four levels of reality — matter, life, thought, and spirit — which ultimately over millennia of time returns to its source, the

---

[7]Teilhard de Chardin, *The Phenomenon of Man*. (Mentor Books: New York, 1961).

Omega Point. This concept follows closely the themes of creation in many religions, namely, Integration, Dis-integration and Re-integration.[7] Aldous Huxley also described four levels — physical, biological, psychosocial, and spiritual — as did Abraham Maslow, but within a more specifically psychological hubris — behavioristic, psychoanalytic, humanistic and transpersonal.[8] Stating that a true science of consciousness will deal with qualities rather than quantities and will be based on shared experiences, physicist Fritzof Capra declared his belief that soul, feelings, and compassion were of the very essence of consciousness.[9] Neuroscientist Karl Pribram and physicist David Bohm have proposed theories that in tandem appear to account for all transcendental experience, paranormal events, and much else besides.[10] As such, they place consciousness within a holotropic frame which since holography embraces all parts of the *whole*, as well as the past, present, and future, seems logical. In a conversation that Dr. Wayne Teasdale, President of the World Parliament of Religions, had with the Dalai Lama in September 1997, His Holiness is quoted as saying: "Consciousness involves absolute, non-dual awareness, unified and not primarily human. This consciousness is animated by an infinitely wise compassion. It is very profound and must bear fruit in some kind of service." Several other scholars have also expanded the parameters of our understanding; but to simplify what at first may seem to be a maze of opinions, let me here describe it from two major perspectives: personal, individual consciousness and evolutionary consciousness.

---

[8]Aldous Huxley, *Evolution in Action*. (Mentor Books: New York, 1953); Abraham Maslow, "Toward a Humanistic Biology. American Psychologist 24, 724-735.

[9]Fritzof Capra, *The Turning Point: Science and Society and the Rising of Culture*. (Bantam Books: New York, 1982).

[10]K. H. Pribram, *What the Fuss Is About In K. Wilber's The Holotropic Paradigm and Other Paradoxes*. (Shambhala: Boulder, CO, 1982); D. Bohm, Wholeness and The Implicate Order. (Routledge and Paul Kegan: London, 1980).

The latter, like the collective consciousness of memory — to which it is a close relative — evolved as a shared property with all humanity. Individual consciousness is said to consist of four states: "waking, dream, sleep, and transcendental." Only in "waking" consciousness are we aware of our thoughts. Yet, if we have learned anything at all from the great scholars and psychotherapists of this and other centuries, we have to be aware of the profound influence of "dream," "sleep," and "transcendental" consciousness on how we perceive reality and, thus, on how we live our lives. In order to understand why, we need to look at the evolution of consciousness itself, that part which we share to some degree with all of humankind and which for ease of understanding, may be compared with the development of a child.

During fetal life and infancy a child is more or less totally dependent on others and is at one with the texture and quality of its environment and sometimes also at its mercy. As a child grows, this dependency lessens as the central nervous and other systems mature, allowing new skills and new awarenesses to be acquired. This leads to new interactive phenomena with the child's environment, giving new meaning to life and existence at each stage of development. Abundant research, including that which I have quoted, shows beyond doubt that the nature and quality of these interactive phenomena convey messages and create expectations about the world outside of *self* which greatly influence later affect and behavior. In other words, during growth and development, while thoughts and *waking* consciousness change, all experience is stored in the memory banks of body, mind, and soul. These memories, though they can be modified, become the bases of belief systems in terms of interpersonal relationships and thus also of behavior. These experiences likewise have a profound effect, if not also a tutoring role, on ego development. This is at the core of how a child perceives him/herself as a separate, independent human being in relation to others. The urge to be free of parental and/or societal regulation and restriction and to exert one's ego independently reaches its peak during adolescence. If the tutoring of experience has been nurturing, then more than likely the turbulent passage of adolescence will give way sooner rather than later to relative calm. If, however, tutoring has been harsh, punishing, and insensitive, the ego is much more likely to take on the combativeness associated with low self-esteem. This can and frequently does lead into the whole spectrum of self-destructive behavior, including addictions as well as dysfunctional, interpersonal behavior, which latter is directed against a world perceived as hostile to self. It is of course when these impasses occur, whether in children, adolescents, or adults, that we invite professional counseling to liberate those suffering from their emotional and behavioral prisons.

> *The purpose of professional counseling is, and should always be, to enable the client to grow into new and healthier awarenesses of self and other. This not only permits healing of scars on the soul, but also allows tolerance, love, and compassion to take up a felt residence in their lives.*[11]

But, the trajectory of the development of individual consciousness is not only beholden to personal experience. It travels with and is influenced by the consciousness that has evolved over millennia from the memories of shared human experience, labeled by Carl Jung as the "Collective Unconscious."

The subject of debate in East and West about its role in dreams and their meaning, as well as in human aspirations and behavior, it has also played a major role in analyses of the myths that not only envelop our origins but which continue to influence our personal and interdependent communal journeys. The world of literature is

---

[11]For additional reading on this subject matter, see Ursula M. Anderson's *The Psalms of Children: Their Songs and Laments. Understanding and Healing the Scars on the Souls of Children.* (She-Bear Publications: Ellicottville, New York, 1997). Pp. 26ff.

full of these marvelous messages. Thanks to their popularization in a television series conducted by Bill Moyers, the writings of Joseph Campbell — particularly his book *The Hero With a Thousand Faces*" — caught the attention and engaged the imagination of many people worldwide.[12] Yet, there have been other scholars and visionaries within, if I may coin an appellation, a psycho-scientific ambience, who have rendered a teleological understanding of it from its beginnings. Pioneered in this century by scientists such as Robert Ornstein and spiritual scholars such as Fr. Bede Griffiths, nevertheless, I will here briefly outline the hypothesis of Ken Wilber who describes the evolution of consciousness in six stages, always, it seems to me, with its primal source in God and in developmental terms that resonate with human development from conception through adulthood. From Stage 1, wherein all creation is at one with its creator, humanity journeys its shared and universal consciousness through the phenomena consequent to its separation from its origin in Creation to its end or *at-one-ment* with its primal source. Stage 2 relates to the sense of separation humankind experienced when expelled from the Garden of Eden and the fears that accompanied the transition from an existence of loving dependency to one wherein this was not palpably present. Language developed in Stage 3, thus allowing description of what was exterior to self by the use of verbal symbols. Language combined with the inner sense of separation from the source of dependent lovingness, which emerged in Stage 2, allowed the concept of blame to form. This was aggrandized during Stage 4 in which *ego* emerged as a driving force. It also coincided with the rapid development of the neo-cortex in the human brain whose function, among others, is rational and logical thought. This not only created within the individual a sense of separate, independent existence, but also provided the means to rationalize and thus intensify the sense of separation of *self from oth-*

---

[12]Bill Moyers' Documentary, P.B.S. Television, USA 1993.

ers. It is within this frame of reference that humankind can create excuses to insist on its individual autonomy and render violence in thought, word and deed on others whom, by being different, it perceives as threats. Stage 5 signals a return to source and, thus, glimmers of an end to the terrors of being separated from it. It is referred to as Trans-Personal consciousness, the awareness that we can reach beyond ourselves to encounter other with love and compassion. This hoped for quality for all humanity has always been at the core of personal spiritual experience and all religions. However, for the past several years, this quality has found a home in the tenets of Trans-Personal Psychology. Stage 5, with its opening to other, is the prelude to the return to source — bringing consciousness full-circle to its beginnings which occurs in Stage 6. Wilber calls this the stage of *supreme consciousness*, wherein, through meditation and compassion for others, we can experience God. It is in this stage that we also encounter the meaning of angels and saints as messengers of love and of eternal universal energy.[13]

It is believed that we carry within us memories of, and the potential to experience all these levels of consciousness. Stages 1 through 4 are mostly experienced within our dream and sleep consciousness from where they influence our waking consciousness. It is Stage 5 that truly calls us to the journey of being divinely human, the transcendence of self to the realization that *other* is also I and that together we can reach *at-one-ment* with God.

If we pay attention to the nuances in Wilber's description of the circular motion of the energies within the evolution of consciousness, it resonates in a profound way with the Genesis story of Creation. Wilber's Stage 1 corresponds with integration, the oneness of humankind in harmony with Creation, which is paradise, the Garden of Eden. His Stage 2 reflects the onset of dis-integration, a

---

[13]Wilber in B. Griffith's, *A New Vision of Reality*. (Templegate Publishers: Chicago, Illinois, 1990

felt or soulful sense of disorder and disconnectedness from the source of creation, that occurred after the Fall — the beginning of exile. The subsequent history of humankind can, I believe, be matched to Wilber's Stages 3 and 4, as well as to the emergence of Stage 5, which despite appearances to the contrary is where humankind may very well be presently situated on its collective journey back to its source.

Stage 3, wherein language developed, can be equated with the scriptural Tower of Babel. It presaged a growing inability to communicate peacefully, giving rise to enmities, misunderstandings, and consequently many genetic and behavioral adaptations to the ensuing stress. Stage 4 represents the emergence of humankind from the bonding that was family and tribal life lived in natural surroundings to the autonomy of the individual and the growing dominance of *ego*, a stage that persists to this day. That it probably has already reached its apogee is reflected in the many signs that we may be at the dawn of Stage 5, such as the concern of stranger for stranger in their extremity as exemplified by those who risk their lives to bring help of all kinds to those suffering because of war, famine, and natural disasters in all parts of the world. More recently, the growing awareness that we are more than the machine that is our body, that we are trinities of body, mind, and soul, is entering into general acceptance and even making dents in the ranks of physicians and health-care professionals. Likewise, the increasing use of alternative methods of healing, rapprochement between religions, and most importantly the awakening to spiritual values rather than the former bondage to organized religion and its hierarchy of control add to these hopeful expectations.

During the millennia it took to evolve through these stages to the present time, there was but one constant and it was *change*. This not only involved how people lived and secured their basic necessities of food, clothing, and shelter, but also how they adapted to their environment. This included their reactions to the threats and presence of danger and disease, as well as how they perceived and related to each other at all levels. Ultimately, of course, these changes involved the genes whose memories of form and function where thereby modified and altered so to ensure survival of the race. Their ability to adapt or, as geneticists would say, mutate has been highly successful, particularly regarding physical integrity and resilience, as evidenced by the multiplication of the human race in numbers so overwhelming that it almost defies human imagination. Into this equation one must also factor the considerable assists that the genetic memories for physical form, function, and survival received from advances in science and even much more so from improvement in the public health and welfare.

But if we look at the changes that more directly influence the quality of soul and its expression in feelings, together with their antecedent thoughts and subsequent behaviors, it is apparent they have not enjoyed the same measure of success. Although the caring soul of humanity sometimes blinds us with its light, nevertheless our world is full of contentions and divisions. Supremacy of ego and distrust of *other* reflects pervasive and worldwide persistence of the genetic memories and other energies that foster these attitudes and behaviors and their fallout transgenerationally. Part of the reason is that health of soul has not received the same intense attention as has health of body. The extent of soul sickness is all too evident in the statistics and stories of violence everywhere, particularly the disturbing increase in violence and abuse done to children *as well as committed by them.* Nevertheless soul remains that still small voice within each and all that whispers and sometimes shouts about its original identity and its yearning to reclaim and proclaim it.

But, because our earthly lives are but a blink on the screen of creation, with our blinkered vision, we may be tempted to be discouraged and to think that we are not moving on to our source but are stuck at a point of no return. After all, history seeks to tell us that despite all the advances in science and technology, our collective behavior as humans has seen little change over the past three to four millennia. In addition, the spiritual teachers who came to remind us of the way to live still await the most of us to listen and to hear. But the evolution of consciousness has been, and remains a long — a very long-journey. Until our beliefs about whom we are as spiritual beings, dependent on each other takes up residence in our souls and in our consciousness, our behavior will not change; but it is *happening*. "The evolution of (wo)man is a gradual ascent through different forms of consciousness to the divine consciousness, which is the ultimate goal of the evolutionary process," said Dom Bede Griffiths, one of the great spiritual leaders of the 20th century, to which I add this ascent is both personal and collective.[14]

Understanding the barriers that impede its blossoming are the gates that we must open to its unfolding. Prominent amongst these are the memories and attitudes that permit abuse and use of others on the false premise that it comes from authority. As co-creators of the earth, and pilgrims in the journey of human consciousness back to its source, we are all equal partners — woman, child, and man. Therefore, no one individual or type of person has the primal right of superiority over others. Yet, as a result of the concept of original sin, this is precisely what has happened. So, let us now enter the labyrinths of discovery of what the theft of original identity has wrought.

---

[14]Bede Griffiths, *Vedanta and Christian Faith*. (Templegate Publishers, Chicago, Illinois, 1991).

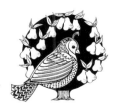

VI

The Consciousness of Woman

OVER THE PAST MANY YEARS, many women have come to consult me as therapist or friend. To my question, "What seems to be the problem?" the answer I receive is usually a variant of "I don't know who I am." This applies to women of varying circumstances and positions: women of all races; women who are homemakers; women who are both professionals and homemakers; those who are married and those who are not; those who are rich and those who are poor; as well as the vast in-between we refer to as the middle class. They cry that they have nothing or want more. Ask most of them to tell you what it is that they are missing or what it is they want more of and the answer will almost always be, "I don't know, but somehow I feel empty."

What they are missing is that sense of *self* and self-*identity* from which flows the dearest of all human gifts, the capacity to be intimate and comfortable with one's self. We tend to think of intimacy as being with another person, but we cannot know intimacy with another person unless we are first in comfortable intimacy with our own self. Attaining such a state requires effort and discipline. In general, the loss of our original identity has blurred our felt sense of connectedness to our source to a point where most of us live behind a mask, some of it woven from transgenerational memories hidden deep within our consciousness and some of it deriving from what we ourselves create to encounter the world in order to survive within it. It is little wonder why many women say, "I don't know who I am."

In the previous chapter, I described how the mythic story of Adam and Eve, and Eve's supposed disobedience, set up all of her descendents as the cause of humanity's problems. In order to prevent any further trouble from Woman, and to establish the hegemony of Man, Woman was made subject to him. This theme pervades the mythology existing within the Judeo-Christian tradition, so much so it serves to instruct us that feminine curiosity and independence that provokes disobedience to male injunctions leads to all kinds of trouble, resulting not only in injury to the feminine spirit, but also, sometimes to her death. Over time, and by virtue of genetic and cultural memories within the collective consciousness, women have been conditioned by the guilt of this cultural/socio-religious history to the point where they continue to give their power away to men.

Of such is the story of Bluebeard. Three sisters and their mother were all quite suspicious of him because of his unusual behavior and his very blue beard and they assumed he was very rich because he lived in a castle. However, when he invited them to go to the woods for a picnic, they camouflaged their fears and went with him. It was the youngest sister who persuaded herself that a man who could be so charming and nice could not be that bad. Thus, when he asked her to marry him, she agreed. One day, shortly after the wedding, Bluebeard informed his wife that he had to go away. He gave her the keys to everything within the castle, including the key to the one room that he forbade her to enter alone. Well, curiosity got the better of her and one day she put the key into the lock of the forbidden room. As she did so, the lock began to bleed. In spite of this warning, she continued to insert the key into the lock and then turned it. As she entered the room, to her horror she beheld the remains of previous wives whose curiosity had also gotten the better of them and who, because of their disobedience to the command of the male, were permanently dispossessed of their identities and their lives by none other than their husband and now hers — Bluebeard.

The important part of the story is the bleeding of the lock. It is a metaphor for the consciousness of woman who knows in her soul that by yielding her *being* and her integrity to the nonsense of male commands — whose intention is control over her, woman surrenders the sacredness of whom she is. In this story, her brothers rescue the young bride from the killing wrath of Bluebeard just in time, but the damage was already done. Forever now, *she*, woman, will know *fear* in her relationship with the male, who has shown her the consequences of disobedience to him and her curiosity, likewise her love for life, has been replaced by a sense of powerlessness. In this story, we see the shadow of Yahweh and the saga of Adam and Eve.

In the Greek mythology of the pre-Christian era, as well as in Eastern mythology and religions, we get a very different idea of the role of the feminine. In the story of Demeter and Persephone, we learn of the yearning of Hades, the male god of the underworld, for the beauty, lovingness, and creativity of Persephone. He realizes that to be *whole* he needs her and, thus, when she is out in the fields one day with her mother Demeter, he steals her. The earth goes into mourning and grieves through fall and winter. During this time, Demeter frantically seeks out her daughter and eventually asks the Sun god to help her find Persephone. He tells Demeter that her daughter is in the underworld, to which Demeter hastens in an attempt to rescue her. The Gods tell Hades that if Persephone has not eaten any of the fruits of the underworld, the daughter must be returned to her mother. Persephone, in her grief over the separation from her mother, has not eaten, but given the idea by other gods, Hades contrives to have a pomegranate pressed to her lips. As she awakens during the journey back to earth, Persephone moistens her lips with her tongue and ingests some of the juice and a seed from the pomegranate. After doing so, Hades tells the gods that she has indeed eaten some of the fruit of the underworld. The gods then decree that Persephone will now have to spend six months in Hades and six months with her mother on earth. During her absence, life on earth had gone into abeyance — it was fall and winter. However, when she returned — bringing joy with her — spring moved in, seeds were planted, and the harvest was gathered in the summer's heat.

In this story, we learn that without the feminine, the male remains incomplete. Thus, we see an immediate dichotomy. In the story about Bluebeard, we are told that unless women obey the male, death will ensue. In other words, women live by permission of the male and on his terms. In the story of Demeter and Persephone, we learn how the male is cold and lifeless without the female and the feminine. Does this conflict and the dilemma it poses sound familiar to those of us living at the dawn of the 21st century? I would say yes, to the nth degree — and, dilemmas always mean stress.

But, is this all? I fear not!

Let us look now at some of the myths that inform us of how women regard other women. On the surface, the Cinderella story is charming. Yet, if we take a closer look, it is the story of how women connive to take away the fulfillment and happiness of other women. In most stories about women and their relationships with each other, happiness and fulfillment are equated not with their own personal growth so much, but with what women have been conditioned to believe is the ultimate prize, which is to have a Prince Charming all of one's own. The message is clear: woman gains identity only by being connected to a man which, if he is indeed Prince Charming, also has *power* and *wealth*. In order to gain her man, Cinderella had to fulfill certain requirements and had, as it were, to run an obstacle course to make herself worthy, since of herself nothing quite fit what was required for her to have her Prince. The plethora of 20th century advertisements mostly coming from the business world informing women of how they can improve on what nature gave them leaves no doubt that women are still conditioned to believe they must work at improving themselves in order to be worthy of the male and his attention. But, when they involve themselves with this, do they win? And, how does it sit with other women?

When I was quite young, I vividly remember the film *Red Shoes*, based on the mythical story of the same name. Moira Shearer, who was the only rival to Margot Fonteyn in the world of the "Royal Ballet" in England, was the star. Readers, you know the story I am sure — the little shoeless orphan who gathered rags of all colors and made herself shoes with the red rags uppermost for the world to see. She exulted in the shoes and loved them because they were a gift of her own creation. One day wandering down a country lane gathering berries, fruits, and nuts to sustain herself, a gilded carriage drew along side and the woman inside leaned out and invited her to get in and go home with her, telling her she would never have to fend for herself again. Once home the first order of business of this woman was to replace the red shoes that the little girl had made for herself with ones made by a master cobbler. At first, she admired them enormously, turning them this way and that, but the more and more she wore these red shoes made by another, the less she could control their activity and the more she moved her feet in them the less she could control their movement. Realizing that she was in great trouble, she tried more than once to get them off and could not because they twirled, and twirled, and twirled and eventually they twirled her into the forest where there lived an executioner.

She begged him to remove her red shoes with his axe, but because they and her feet were now as it were glued together, he could not do so without cutting off her feet, to which in her desperation she agreed. Thus she became crippled and had to live the rest of her life dependent on others. The message is loud and clear. Her own creativity and her own power were stolen by another woman who thought she knew what was best for her, thus forever taking away her ability to truly become her own creation — her own *self*.

Yet, looking once again at how woman is regarded in Greek mythology and Eastern religions, we discover that it is woman, the feminine who lives in the hidden place that everyone, man and woman, knows, yet few have seen or touched. It is the feminine who can show us what is right for the soul; *she is the eternal intuition, the connection with the eternal and with the creator.* Indeed, one of the most widespread archetypical personifications in the world is that of the wise old woman, the *Crone*. She it is, who is the feed to the root of an entire instinctual system. There are many names for her, including, *the heroine/warrior, the great father/mother, and the one who knows.*

Whatever happened to her? Is what happened to her and her absence in the lives of women — the root of woman's loss of self-identity? I believe so.

The great privilege of life and living is becoming and being who we are and who we were born to be. It is the endless search for the Holy Grail, the part that is missing that if found will make us whole. There is endless mythology around the Holy Grail, many people still believing that it is the chalice used by Christ at the Last Supper. Other scholars believe that it is the platter on which Christ laid the bread he later broke and gave to his apostles at the Last Supper. History has it that Joseph of Aramethia, who provided the tomb for Christ, brought he platter to Glastonbury in England, which is the center of the legends that surround the Holy Grail, King Arthur,

The Round Table, Queen Guinevere, Sir Lancelot, and Merlin. In the Judeo-Christian tradition, bread and wine are at the symbolic center of worship and represent the nourishment of Life by Eternal Energy, the Great and Holy Spirit, the one GOD. Thus, those who seek the Holy Grail are seeking not the chalice or the platter on which the bread was laid, but the Bread and Wine of Life itself, which is to know within our own beings wholeness, love, hope, and oneness with Creation and to be without fear. So if we as women have had our power to pursue the grail within our own lives stolen from us by men, and blemished by women who resent women who have taken the road to self empowerment, then *whom are we? What do we seek and what are the consequences of our agony?*

And, who and what is the Feminine?"

Across all major religions, there is Trinity. Woman, too, is a trinity. She is first the birther; secondly, the nurturer; thirdly, she is the crone, the wise older woman, the one who knows, who intuits, and who loves unconditionally. The threads that bind this trinity are consciousness and memory.

From about 7000 BCE, people of Southern Europe were agriculturists, matriarchal, and goddess worshipping, taking from the earth what was needed for life and returning with reverence what was no longer needed. As villages were built, many shrines to the goddess were also built. Goddess and woman, giving birth, nurturing, and strengthening was the pivot of their lives. Those who blessed the mother/goddess gathered at sacred wells and springs, some which continue to exist today, and are becoming increasingly popular as places of historical interest. Those villages that have been excavated show no signs of weaponry and no signs of animal slaughter. In these ancient burial places, there are many representations of the goddess, *"mother of all,"* with wide hips for birthing and many breasts to nourish symbolically all of earth's children, and women, the embodiment of the goddess, seem to have been treated with great honor and respect.

If we allow ourselves a swift journey from that point in history until now, one may ask, "What have we allowed to be done to our role, as woman giving birth, nurturing and strengthening our creations as well as nurturing and strengthening Mother Earth?" It seems as though in the dark ages, men learned to fear the spiritual and sexual being of women and they found ways of co-opting what they feared to use as power against them. Thus, by the time of the Industrial Revolution in Europe just three centuries ago, men were perceived as the prime movers of all that was central to the creation of money and power; women and children were exploited terribly and concern for them was at a premium. Indeed in 1911 in England, Winston Churchill, who many believe was one of the greatest men who ever inhabited Mother Earth, helped to found the first National Health Insurance scheme in England, all of whose benefits were directed toward the working man. This simply reflected the attitude of the time that saw the exploitation of women and children who were contributing as much, if not more, to the national wealth as were the working men as being of no concern. The suffragette movement in England starting in the early part of the 20th century sought to bring attention to the desperate plight of women and children, for women were not only excluded from voting for the people who had power and used it against them, but they were excluded from any kind of surcease from the ill effects of their usage by men in the factories and in the home. In the United States of America it took women of great courage and determination like Rose Hawthorne, the daughter of Nathaniel Hawthorne, Julia Lathrop, and others who lobbied Congress for years to get a bill passed that provided a governmental office to promote attention to the needs of mothers and children. Although the Children's Bureau was established in 1912, its functions were mostly advisory until in 1935 President Franklin Delano Roosevelt signed the Social

Security Act under Title 5 of which monies were set aside to pro-vide direct health services to mothers and children. If one has kept up with the activities of those involved with the welfare of children, such as the Children's Defense Fund, the Academy of Pediatrics, and others, it is clear that from the beginning it has been a struggle to have mothers and children included in legislation that will pro-vide for their basic health and social needs. Most thoughtful people, and in increasing numbers, believe that the experience of pregnan-cy and childbirth is the most important part of the whole of human experience regardless of gender. Yet in our society this is given little or no attention, and, in fact, our way of birthing works against it. For example, about a half-century ago, bureaucratic decisions were made to build large maternity hospitals because hospital births were believed to be the safest. Subsequently, it was assumed, incorrectly, that hospital delivery was responsible for the lowering of maternal and infant mortality rates. However, if one examines the trends of maternal infant, and child mortality rates over the last 100 years in most developed nations, it is obvious that the lowering of the mor-tality rates coincided with implementation of universal education and improved social conditions. While no one can argue with the aim of having all women delivered of a healthy infant, we have to look as what hospital-based deliveries and technology are doing to the spirituality and emotionality of childbirth. For starters, hospital delivery mandated that infants be taken from their mother immedi-ately after birth, turned upside down, and slapped "to promote their first breath." Coming from the relative protection of the womb, this first encounter with the outside world can only be classed as violent.

Coincident with the increase in hospital births was the rise of the specialty of Obstetrics and Gynecology which until recently was male dominated. Is it because women are regaining the sense that they have given the power of their reproduction away to men that we now have a thrust toward home-based deliveries with midwives rather than obstetricians in attendance? Writing in the August 1991

issue of *Aisling*, a journal published in Ireland, Carmel Duffy, a well
-known Irish archaeologist, observed that today childbirth is a man-
aged affair. She states, however, that if a woman is to give birth, she
must open up absolutely, physically, mentally and spiritually, and let
go, so that the new life can come into being. If held on to and man-
aged, the deep spiritual meaning of the experience is hobbled. She
further states that during each of her seven pregnancies, she was
coerced by her physician not to have her child delivered at home,
but to have it delivered in the hospital. She states that her failure to
comply led physicians to intimidate and frighten her into doing
things their way. I believe, as she does, that women should not be
afraid to experience and exercise the power that the Great Spirit of
life has entrusted to them by making them mothers. In this context,
I believe that each woman should ask the meaning of all procedures
that are currently carried out during pregnancy. A recent study, for
example, showed that sonograms do not improve the immediate
outcome of pregnancy. Apart from the expense of these procedures
and that they are doing nothing to improve the immediate outcome
of pregnancy, one must ask what are they doing in the long term to
unborn children. Years ago, I suspected that ultrasonography, which
at that time, and I believe still is, considered by some to be a non-
invasive procedure, is actually a highly invasive procedure. The
high-frequency waves that go through a woman's body in order to
give an image of the fetus are like so many fine-tuned ultra-sharp
knives which produce images when they impact on masses of different density, in this case the fetus. Sonograms are done during pregnancy at the time of migration of nerve cells from the notochord to
the brain. What is this invasion of high-frequency waves doing to
the orderly migration of cells? I believe that it may be scrambling it.
I believe it may be interfering with the migration of the cells to their
appropriate places in the brain. Then the question becomes, does
this have any relation to the rising epidemic of learning and behavioral problems in children? Thus, is it indirectly contributing to the
pandemic of violence in our society? I think these are questions of

profound societal impact and importance, and research should be developed immediately to give us the answers. Also, at about 28 weeks of pregnancy, women are given the glucola test, which is a test to discover whether or not they are at risk for pregnancy induced diabetes. For several hours after taking 50 grams of glucola, a fetal heart will beat more than 140 times per minute, often so fast it is uncountable. Further, what is this doing to sensitize the whole endocrine system of the unborn child to future sugar imbalances, and what is it doing to create memories in the brain for the rush of sugar from drugs and alcohol because electrochemical messages in the cells of our bodies leave memories that remain there for always? Addicts will tell us that what they are addicted to is the memory and pleasure of the rush that their addiction gives them.

Combining all of this with the importance of loving touch and contact at and immediately following birth elsewhere referred to hauls into question hospitals as birthing places. For sure, labor and delivery in high-risk pregnancies should occur in a place where the resources necessary to bring about safe delivery for mother and child are available. This means they should take place in a hospital. However, what about the 95% of normal deliveries? Should they not take place in a nurturing environment where the mother has known love and, hopefully, where the child has been conceived in love? For many years, there has been in place an efficient three-layered approach to the management of all pregnancies. Surely we can continue to plug into those fine systems that were created a quarter of a century or more ago, so that unexpected difficulties can be handled at a moment's notice and the mother transferred to a place where she can be safely delivered. As birthers, women have much to ask themselves in terms of the power they have given away and which they need to reclaim over the birthing process. Indeed, one has to wonder about the long-term effects of depression and anxiety that result from women having had as it were the natural approach to childbirth taken away from them, a question not to be answered quickly, but one that surely deserves attention. In this regard, although there has been an understandable outcry over insurance companies limiting hospital stay for delivery to 24-hours, based of course on financial considerations and the historic trend to devalue the health of women and children by saving on their needs first, the move could have positive outcomes— only, but only, if women see and seize the opportunity to lobby for home delivery with qualified midwives. We will see, but meanwhile we should not hold our breath.

Concerning women as nurturers, beginning with the basics, what about breast-feeding? Have women been seduced by the Madison Avenue advertising techniques and the blitz of the baby food companies? Abundant research has confirmed that not only does breast-feeding allow bonding to occur between the mother and child, but it provides the best food the child can have in the first few months of its life. Human milk not only has all of the minerals, proteins, carbohydrates, and fats, in proper proportions for a human child, it carries the immune factors that no bottle can ever provide. Alas, the baby food companies took over to the tune of enormous profits, but the fact remains that no matter how you try to humanize cow's milk, cow's milk was made for baby cows, and no matter how you alter it to try and make it like human milk, it can never be human milk. Likewise, baby foods prepared and canned in factories have taken away the joy of preparing food as nurturance for children, much better by far prepared in the kitchen of the home than in a factory. The messages to women are not so subtle. As nurturers, they are considered inadequate. And then, throughout the childhood years, high-tech advertising instructs mothers on how to feed and clothe their children and school systems tell them what their children should learn without much reference to the nurturing of their souls and the balance that should exist between their minds, bodies, and souls. These, and other issues, impact on how women are denied the chance of being nurturers, not only to their children and families, but to themselves — a situation to which other factors also contribute.

There is an eternal conflict between pursuing a sense of well-being through self-identity versus a sense of well-being through the relationships we form. In general, women find identity in relationships. However, the so-called woman's revolution of the last several decades has invited, or should I say pushed, women to find identity outside of relationships within the family and the home. By working outside of the home, women have to seek self-identity within that environment which is predominately a male way of finding meaning. Many women who work outside of the home feel in the depth of their souls a kind of emptiness and some believe, as I do, that this is why creative women in particular suffer from chronic depression. From earliest times, the feminine has added gentleness and wholeness to the human experience. Frequently gentleness is partially absent, if not totally, from the work environment. When this happens, there is a silence within the soul. In order to succeed in the work environment, women almost have to lose touch with their femininity. A man in his own world expects to receive from a woman emotional and practical support in his pursuit of *identity* through his work. When women are in the workplace, they also need, but seldom receive, the same emotional and practical support from the men in their lives. Furthermore, when women are in this conflictual situation, the shadow side of striving for one's personal identity emerges. The shadow side is felt when one fails to attain the success one expected and/or the sense of achievement and well-being that is often projected to it. This, alas, is not an uncommon occurrence among women in the workplace. Shadow creates a sense of failure, and failure leads to guilt. Guilt creates fear and fear is the footprint of depression and anxiety. This, of course, impacts in a heavy and negative way on a woman's ability to find identity through relationships which is her natural way of doing so. So women are not only put into a bind when they work outside the home seeking identity, but given that their natural instinct is to find identity through relationships they have the double consequence of shame and guilt if they perceive themselves as not succeeding in either role. Women come into this world with a psyche imprinted with archetypal impressions. When there is conflict, women mourn for their lost femininity which they sense in their souls. This conflict, and its manifold fallout, is of very real concern in terms of women's sense of well-being. It gives rise to identity, emotional, and personality problems which contribute in great measure to the stress underlying all women's health issues. Woman as nurturer must think in terms of nurturing herself as well as her children and her spouse. This brings me back to the first point I made — that unless women identify whom they are as women, and unless they can be intimate with that and themselves, then true intimacy with another can never be achieved.

Women also need to be nurturers to other women. Are the stories of Cinderella and Red Shoes still alive and well today? I believe they are. In the many journals that I read, in recent years I have been very dismayed at the stories of young women in training to be physicians who are not only subjected to the hazing of male medical students, but have to run the gauntlet of what is perceived to be competition for these Prince Charmings on the part of other female health workers in more traditional professions. For example, we all love nurses, but there is a particular energy that goes between nurses and female medical students, and young female physicians and indeed older ones as well. Endless articles have been written recently about it, the genesis of which I believe lies in the Cinderella story, every woman wanting the same Prince Charming, but I believe it may be also deeper than that. Then again, how many times does one hear of women in high positions having difficulty finding a female secretary, not because there is anything the matter with the high-achieving woman, but just on instinct and impulse when a woman hears that her boss is going to be a woman, she will frequently bow out of the picture even though she hasn't even met the woman who is going to be her boss. The heavier the reputation a woman has, the more creative she is, the more paranoia she creates in women who have not traveled her journey. A woman who embraces the ultimate in following her brilliance and her desire to find identity not only through her personal and professional achievements but in her relationships *is* most truly a great heroine, the feminine archetype of Joseph Campbell's concept of hero/heroine. It is one of the most difficult of human journeys in our culture. Many books have been written about how women are conditioned to think about other women — "Mothers and Daughters" and "The Cinderella Story," are two examples among many others. A profound question that hovers over the inability of women to accept and be nurturing toward other women is that, although they outnumber men, they are perceived and referred to as a minority. This then sets up those who refuse to accept a minority role as target for defamation by those who do. Does the old adage divide and conquer apply to us women? I think the answer is obvious. Does this not have profound implications for women's identity?

Certainly it does.

As women, through the cycles in our own bodies, we are in touch with the cycles of the earth and the universe. It is believed that the chaotic order of the universe would fall apart if one tiny part of its consciousness was to be disturbed. So, too, with women. When, in the deepest part of our feminine soul, we are in conflict about who we are and what our roles are, our bodies and minds suffer. Without attempting to oversimplify a very complicated phenomenon, nevertheless, the number of women who suffer from Premenstrual Stress Syndrome (P.M.S.) is astounding. It is now so prevalent that, when the powers that be were considering what to include and not include in the new DSM-IV, which is the Diagnostic Statistical Manual for Psychiatric Disorders, there was a great debate about whether or not to include premenstrual stress syndrome as a pathological entity. Fortunately, there was wisdom around when this issue was being discussed and a task force of women was established to consider it. But, had Premenstrual Stress Syndrome been included in the DSM IV, 70% of women would thereby have been labeled as psychiatrically disturbed. Just imagine what this would have done to the self-esteem of women and how it would have overflowed in a negative way into the collective consciousness. Compromise was achieved by including it according to the severity of its disabling symptoms. However, the basic question is why do so many women have PMS syndrome?

Thinking about this for a moment invites one to think about all that is perceived about woman as nurturer and what it has done to the feminine psyche. Years and years ago, I had a very dear friend who was the director of social work at a large hospital; when we were talking in a semi-counseling session, she said, "I just feel that I am schizophrenic." She was, of course, not schizophrenic in the clinical sense of the word, but what she was referring to was the constant conflict and confusion about whom she was as a woman living in a man's world and trying at the same time to maintain and retain emotional relationships with herself, her family, and with the rest of the world. Does that cause stress? Of course, it does, and when stress is present, dysfunction ensues.

The third part of the *trinity* of woman, is that of the *crone*, the wise, older woman. The woman who endures and who responds to the feminine within her soul during the endurance test that is her life does become the crone. Although many women yield to the temptation to give their power away to men, particularly men of money and power, there are many women who instinctively know and who come to know by experience that money, power, and authority are masks. These women realize at some point or other in their lives that true power lies within one's self and that each of us is a part of the expression of the Great Creator, the great, divine, creative spirit. This divine spark lies at the core of our being and when we relinquish the pursuit of knowing, nurturing and loving that deepest part of ourselves which is our eternal spirit we lose our comfort and our meaning. When women reclaim it, they are on the road to wisdom — to becoming the crone, the wise, older woman, the one who has the answers of peace and acceptance to life, its joys and its tragedies.

I believe that the tragedies of life result mostly from our sense of separation from the source of our being, which is *love* and *creation*. This separation can be self-inflicted as well as being the consequence of what life does to us. In passing, I would like to make reference to what I think is a common misconception about creating our own reality. This is an often-talked-about topic these days and I think it has some danger in terms of laying guilt on those who seem unable to control the realities of their lives. In fact, we often have little or no control over the things that occur in our lives. For example, we have little or no control over natural disasters or accidents nor of what happens to other people. However, we do in great measure have control and can exert control over our reactions to these events. It is when we realize that we do have the inner wisdom to monitor *our* reactions that we begin to be in touch with the wise older woman, the crone deep within ourselves. Those who have moved through these times of trial respond to the invitation of the infinite to grow beyond circumstance to the knowing of the great darkness, which is *infinity*, that lies beyond the illumination of suffering, but, this is never easy and in some instances impossible.

For most of the world's women, moving through their dispossession of self and self-identity to possession of self and self-identity remains an elusive dream. Evidence of their continued and frequent brutalization almost staggers the imagination. For example, just before the fourth *U.N. World Conference on Women* held in September 1995 in Beijing, China, Amnesty International proposed four urgent lines of action to secure equal justice and human rights for women. They were

- Expose the worldwide scandal of escalating sexual torture and sustained abuse of women in both peace and war.

- Confront government indifference and complicity in encouraging the abuse of women around the world.

- Publicize the brutal violations against individual women and step up urgent actions on their behalf.

- Press government authorities to promote women's basic human rights and petition for the swift delivery of real protection for women at risk.[1]

The report went on to say that women have become, among other things, the invisible victims of the 1990s: the primary casualties of war; 80% of the world's refugees; and the target of human rights violations on a horrifying scale. Amnesty's 135-page report on the global condition of women's human rights, their graphic case studies and the damning country reports, have already begun to expose what is nothing less than a worldwide scandal.

In wars and civil conflicts, women are often targeted for reprisal killings and singled out for rape and sexual assault which, increasingly, has become a weapon of war. The discriminatory treatment of women in many countries means they are more likely to suffer abuses that are not treated as crimes and that they will be far less likely to have these abuses exposed. These abuses are legion: women are raped in custody, are forced to take virginity tests by police, are flogged for violating dress codes, and even risk being stoned to death for "sexual offenses." The abuse of women remains not only largely hidden but also largely ignored by world governments. Many governments, who only recently adopted the "U.N. Declaration on the Elimination of all Forms of Violence Against

---

[1]Taken from a memorandum to all Amnesty Members from William F. Schultz, Executive Director (June 22, 1995).

Women," are responsible for appalling and increasing levels of violence against them. Women who have experienced sexual torture and other abuse pay the price with lifelong psychological damage, serious physical injury, pregnancy, disease, and death. In her memoir *Do They Hear You When You Cry*, Fauzia Kassindja, a native of Togo in West Africa, gives a human face to the torture of the blood-soaked ritual of Kakia — otherwise known as female genital mutilation which is widely practiced throughout the world. She recounts that four women spread your legs wide apart, hold you down, and scrape away all your woman parts. After forty days, you are "reborn" for your husband and delivered to his house. Thankfully, women are finding a voice to protest and bring to an end this barbaric torture. In other countries where low wages, long hours, and sexual harassment are typical of their working conditions, some women have found the strength to organize and begin changing their situation, despite threats of firing, blackmail, and even death. These abuses have a tremendous fallout not only in the personal suffering of women, but on their children, families, and ultimately on society.

Albeit with an emphasis on Western women, their causative relationship to physical illness has been admirably addressed by Dr. Christine Northrup in her best-selling book *Women's Bodies; Women's Wisdom*. Citing "Toxic People" from past or present, "Toxic Thoughts, Attitudes and Ideas" about "a woman's place" as central to most physical illness, she documents incontrovertable evidence of how women are ignored, neglected, or at best patronized by the medical establishment.[2] While they account for half of all visits to physician's offices, women receive 83% of all prescriptions for anti-depressant drugs — surely a brush-off for real problems of soul that results in three-quarters of all patients in mental hospitals being women. Is this to be wondered at when half of all women and chil-

---

[2]Christine Northrup, *Women's Bodies, Women's Wisdom*. (New York: Bantam Books, 1994).

dren in the US are victims of domestic violence, and that the number of women who die as a result of spousal and family violence in any five-year period in the USA equals or is in excess of all American fatalities in the Vietnam War? The latter have a monument to their memory in Washington, D.C., but there are no monuments to these women, only the transgenerational continuance of what was done to them as memories in the individual consciousness of their children and the collective consciousness of society, which, of course, serves to perpetuate the problems.

Children of battered women have significantly more developmental, learning, and behavioral problems than do children who have not experienced this trauma. I have no doubt that if this is put into the context of memory and consciousness, these sequelae are due to changes in the energy patterns of memory that ultimately impact negatively on the genes that influence and/or control these functions. The pivotal role of the mother's emotional health and stability in the health and welfare of her children has been abundantly documented. Indeed, the authors of a study carried out in New Zealand and reported in *Pediatrics* in 1984 concluded that the *major* contributing factor to problems in child rearing was maternal depression brought on by negative family-life events.[3] Other research has shown time and again that even the smallest of infants are so highly attuned to the moods of their parents, especially those of their mother, that when mother-child interactions are interfered with by the mother's depression, their infants respond by showing sadness, social withdrawal, and helplessness, the latter being an early sign of learning impairment.

Yet, despite the abundance of knowledge we have about the importance of maternal health of body, mind, and soul, not only for themselves but also for their children, so far the emphasis has been

---

[3]D.M. Ferguson et al., "Relationship of Family Life Events, Matenal Depression and Child Rearing Problems," in *Pediatrics* 73, 6, June 1984.

on physical health while the beat goes on with the denouement of emotional and spiritual well-being. A study conducted by Lois Weiss, Ph.D. of the University at Buffalo Graduate School of Education, and Michelle Fine of CUNY Graduate School revealed what the authors described as a horrific picture of women's lives saturated with serious domestic violence.[4] Ninety-two percent of white female respondents said that serious domestic violence was directed against them, their mothers, and/or sisters either in their birth households or in later relationships. Serious domestic violence was defined as battering intended to cause serious physical injury. By comparison, 62% of black female respondents reported similar levels of violence in their lives. Furthermore, while black women were not secretive either in personal interviews or group sessions, white women spoke openly only in private sessions. The authors observed that one way white women maintain their racial difference is to cultivate the popular cultural image of the perfectly functioning white nuclear family.

In an article in the *Toronto Globe and Mail* of July 17, 1996 titled "When the First Man Turns You Away," it was poignantly stated that,

> *"If the one man who is supposed to provide you (the female) with unconditional love withholds affection it becomes a deeply ingrained habit to wonder what is intrinsically wrong with you; to wonder if others can see it as well and then fight, inexhaustibly, to either prove them wrong or prove them right — but at least prove you're worth attention. Thus, abusive relationships become the norm because you know what to expect from them — the familiarity assures you that you belong in them. And echoing what I have heard so often from my clients," she added, "Mothers loved us deeply but not enough to see the damage being done and not*

---

[4]Lois Weiss and Michelle Fine, *The Unknown City: The Lives of Poor and Working Class Young Adults.* (Beacon Press: New York, 1998).

enough to choose us over him. Brothers perceive this also and prac-
tice the callousness they've been taught by their male role models
— expecting to be loved, nurtured and oh, yes, even adored —
regardless their behavior because, well, isn't this the way their
mothers (loved) endured their fathers."

In this regard, I have often been made keenly aware of how men compartmentalize their relationships with women: extending respect and devotion to their mothers versus disrespect and often abuse to all others. It is a theme brilliantly and often humorously addressed by Dr. Rafael Lopez-Corvo in his book *God Is a Woman*, in which he explores the power that women exert over men.[5] He argues that the violence toward women is based on man's eternal longing for his mother and envy of woman's ability to bear children sentiments I myself have frequently heard expressed by men. He suggests that women should search for their own identity, a pursuit that I heartily endorse, and he suggests they should find a place where God could be a woman. I do believe that when the collective consciousness reaches a critical point as a result of women discovering, encountering and living their identity, then reverence for the feminine will be established and restored. Perhaps, then, this will become the place and the point in time where God will be a woman, but meanwhile, it is quite evident that we have far to travel to that expectantly golden world.

Statistics in the U.S. reveal that battering accounts for 1 out of 5 women seeking medical care, as well as the reason for up to 35% of their visits to hospital emergency rooms. Yet, if one looks only for trauma in these situations, the vast majority of battered women will be overlooked. Violence in the home often manifests as anxiety, depression, chemical dependency, chronic headaches, sleeping and eating disorders, a wide variety of somatic complaints, as well as sui-

---

[5]Rafael Lopez-Corvo, *God Is a Woman*. (Northvale, NJ: Jason Aronson, 1997).

cide attempts. The dynamic in battering and violence is power and control over the victim which is often reinforced by the victim's fear of reprisals should they report it to the authorities. It is common knowledge that at the scene of domestic assaults, victims often beg police not to arrest their batterer, and in courts women frequently demand that charges against their tormentors be dropped. The tragedy is that most women in these situations realize that no matter what they do, they are in danger of their lives. Most abusers justify their disgusting behavior by blaming it on some perceived flaw in their victims; in so doing, they hold their victim responsible for the violence. "Look what you made me do" is the statement an abuser frequently makes after a violent episode.

Fifty percent (50%) of all women murdered in the U.S. are killed by a current or former partner, Yet, if we look for a concerted and focused effort to halt this physical, emotional, spiritual, and transgenerational carnage, there is none. Rather, there are a few programs scattered here and there that jab at one or another aspect of the overall problem. A few of these are educational in the sense that they seek to change attitudes prevalent in society that identifies women as sub-human or at best not in any way equal to men. By depersonalizing women, such beliefs make it easier to be abusive of them; after all, hitting a peer or one's equal is so rare it makes news! Such depersonalization is fostered and promoted by the lucrative pornography industries all over the world that portray mutilation and torture of women and children as a male sport. Sexual fantasies and stories of women being kidnapped, sodomized, mutilated, and left to die by men who show no remorse are creeping on to the Internet. That sexual fantasy turns into sexual abuse is still being debated, though one wonders why. As Catherine MacKinnon, a law professor and a leader in advocacy for women's rights and author of *Only Words*, states: "Writing and reading pornography are in themselves acts of violence." Further evidence of the dispensability of women and children is reflected in a recent UNICEF bulletin which stated that in the so-called Third World in 1997, an estimated six million or more children were starving and because of discrimination against women and their low status, leading to poor nutrition, millions more were born prematurely with all of its attendant risks many others were born with crippling conditions.

Within all of this, it is easy to discern the legacy of Eve. Blame continues to be placed on women for the problems of men, and because of her inferiority, woman is subject to his power, control, and usage. At this point, it is well to keep in mind what has already been addressed — that the tale of Creation and the expulsion from the Garden of Eden are in scriptural texts written by men and only about four thousand years or less ago, which in terms of human evolution is a mere blink in the march of time. The prodigious accomplishments and research of the brilliant scholar, archeologist, and linguist Dr. Marija Gimbutas, who recently died, leave no doubt that prior to Old Testament times, women were revered as the soul of creation. Indeed, woman was the goddess on whom all life depended and from whom all life flowed.[6]

As to why such a drastic change in the relationship of male and female occurred, in addition to the possibilities previously mentioned, it is not beyond feasibility that within the context of the evolution of human consciousness, the emergence and dominance of *ego* could well have caused male rebellion against the power of the female. Her power was vested in her fecundity, and it was this that men sought to control and continue to do so. Over time, it is conceivable that the biology of the male and his greater physical strength married to his ego succeeded in making him dominant. Once able to intimidate the female verbally and physically, it was a short step to casting his dominance in stone and this was cleverly

---

[6]See Marija Gimbutas, *The Bronze Age Cultures of Central and Eastern Europe.* (Mouton: The Hague, 1965); *The Language of the Goddess.* (San Francisco: Harper, 1991) and *Civilization of the Goddess.* (San Francisco: Harper, 1991).

accomplished by invoking the imprimatur of the Goddess herself, clothed now in a male image. Armed with this permission, male hegemony straddled and strangled the feminine by assuming control over the source of her power, which is creation, and so it has been since the days wherein the Old Testament was written. We live in an era where this is all too visible. Men not only make laws about the outcome of sexual encounters between themselves and women, but laws that punish them if they disobey their dictates.

It is evident that once blame on women and their subservience to men was codified in religious texts, which incidentally are curiously silent about male responsibility for the consequences of sexual activity, the stage was set for their exploitation. Proclaiming God, who was *now* male, as the source of their authority, men passed laws and organized society to ensure their dominance. Women were denied rights to property and self-realization and considered chattels to be used, abused, and controlled by men who exercised total power over them. At the core was the loss of ownership of their own bodies and souls, a fact that in the 19th century made the great lady Florence Nightingale observe, "Today is my 30th birthday and I am glad that those years wherein a woman owns nothing, not ever her own soul, are now behind me." She was, of course, mis-taken; for, in spite of her great accomplishments, not only in nursing, but in concern for social issues, she continued to face and battle put-downs from men, much less gifted than she until the end of her life.

While the scriptural story of Adam and Eve is the prototype of what has been the "norm" over the past several millennia, and which still continues, is it to be wondered that in societies regarded as being religious in the sense of church controlling the masses, the abuse of women and children is endemic? An article in the February 22, 1998 issue of the *Manchester Guardian Weekly* addressed what is happening in Poland. The headline stated: "Women in Poland Lose Habit of Submission." To address the epidemic of domestic violence, the Center for Human Rights was established in Warsaw just two years ago by Ursula Nowakowska. Her aim is to drive into the public domain an issue, which from time immemorial was considered a private, family matter. A hotline established for victims is being hassled by men who call for an end to this meddling in "their" private affairs. Most significantly, and recently, a government office for women and children has been replaced by an office for family affairs and is headed by an archconservative male. And, yet, a year or so ago, a Polish Pope revealed his conversion to the plight of women by calling on men to be more involved with their families and the loving raising of their children. Evidently, that message has yet to reach his homeland! In revealing his conversion, the Pope said, "… When one looks at the great process of women's liberation, the journey has been a difficult and complicated one, … substantially a positive one, even if it is still unfinished."[7] Those of us who remember and felt the pain of how, on his first visit to the USA, Pope John Paul II crudely and rudely dismissed the women who reverently asked for a voice in the church, can only point to his conversion as what is possible when one becomes enlightened.

The systematic erosion of the feminine and abuse of her identity is deeply embedded in the memory and soul of every woman. Therefore, when they say, "I don't know who I am," they are proclaiming what the loss of feminine identity has wrought, at least since the time of Genesis. Additionally, on an individual level this injury to collective consciousness interplays with personal experience to create the *power-less-ness* at the center of so much anguish and morbidity experienced by women.

However, this is not all.

The male who abuses the female does violence to his own soul and, in so doing, further distances himself from his original identity of *at-one-ment* with his Creator. Furthermore, by witnessing vio-

---

[7]Pope John Paul II, *Easter Address to Priests*, 1997.

lence in the place where there should be love and respect, horrendous injuries are inflicted on the souls of children, whose memories persist forever. These memories and the anxiety, depression, and despair that violence generates become the precursors of its transmission from generation to generation. These are the scars on the souls of humankind — men, women and children — everywhere. Their healing requires far more than the bandages we presently apply to them. In fact, what is needed is nothing less than a radical transformation of our attitudes and a rekindling of respect for "She," without whom there would be no men. In so doing, humankind must seek to recreate the holy and wholesome alliance of male and female and, thus, send the light of this *one-ness* as a message of *hope* and *love* to humankind. First, however, we must be about educating all children, male and female, about the beauty and the spirit of the feminine. Even if we could start now, it will take two to three generations before the critical level of changed memories and their energies become perceptible. This endeavor can only be enhanced and enriched by our understanding of what children themselves have been subjected to in the pursuit of wealth and status for men — a territory we will now explore.

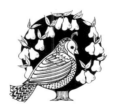

VII

Children in History

Their Use and Expendability
& The Emergence of Concerns
for Their Physical Health

THE WORLD OF CHILDREN is filled with contradictions. There are uncountable numbers of unwanted children. Millions who have been abandoned, eke out an existence on the streets of some of the major cities of the world, where they roam in bands seeking to steal for subsistence, thus terrorizing the citizenry and, in turn, being terrorized and even gunned down by law enforcement agencies who perceive them as human garbage.

In the United States of America, the land of plenty, in 1994 one-quarter of a million children were homeless. In the same year, over half a million children were in foster care and the possibility of adoption for most of them was an impossible dream.

Yet, obversely, people expend themselves and their energies in fundraising activities to find cures for childhood diseases and not always because they are parents of an afflicted child. Others volunteer love and time to make summer camps and other activities available to poor children, as well as those with chronic and life-threatening diseases. When a child is in danger, no effort is spared for its rescue. When a child dies, whether close or far, relative, friend or stranger, many of us grieve. Similarly, with great fanfare, government underwrites programs, amounting to billions of dollars, to ensure that all children are immunized against physical disease when, in fact, immunization levels are the highest on record and statistics tell us that physical diseases are no longer the killers of children.

The "killing fields" of children in the so-called developed nations — where development, in fact, largely reflects their technology — are diseases of the soul. Abuse — verbal, emotional, physical, sexual, and spiritual, as well as a concomitant lack of love and respect, married to neglect and abandonment, are the diseases and dysfunctions that beg our attention. Yet, there has been no great government program to ensure immunization against these killers nor any fanfare to declare the devastatingly personal and transgenerational nature of their effects. Their origins reside within the theft of their original identity and the permission so granted to those who stole it to devalue children as unique spiritual beings.

Practical concern for the consequent carnage began when a few compassionate souls turned their attention toward reducing the appallingly high infant mortality. While these multilayered efforts have over the last two centuries been enormously successful, at the outset they were in fact strange bedfellows with the concomitant and unconscionable exploitation of women and children in the furtherance of the money economy that then as now was the breadbasket of Western culture. Holding up the mirror to these contrasts, particularly in regard to infant mortality, is a holotropic revelation, the whole contained within this fragment of human history, the struggle between greed and compassion, good and evil, in essence the on-going drama of the genesis story of creation. As such it has much to teach us about the memories and consciousness that influence and indirectly direct our beliefs about children and our attitudes and behavior toward them, most of which can be summarized within the rubric of "a child's place."

In the U.S. in 1900, the infant mortality rate (IMR) was approximately 130, which means that out of every 1000 infants born that year, 130 died before their first birthday. In 1915, it was 99.9, and in 1993, it was 8.2. Despite this spectacular achievement, the USA actually ranked 21st among the nations of the world, Japan being number 1 with an IMR of 4.4. Similar success in improving infant survival is part of the history of most European countries. For example, in Great Britain in 1870 the IMR was 153, in 1915 was 110, and in 1993 was 6.5. Hidden within these dramas are the intertwining origins of much that we presently take for granted in the realms of health and human services, particularly community and public health. It is rather like a historical road map wherein roads leading from several distant and apparently unrelated sites have intersected and eventually connected to build the highway along which we presently travel.

Thus, remote as it may seem, improvement in infant survival and our current fascination with immunology both had their origins in the 13th century. It was during this century that the money economy, which ever since has been the lubricant for national growth and expansion, was first established. It flowed from the commerce and industry that flourished in the new towns and cities of 13th century Europe whose origins lay within the political scientific and social changes that took place in late medieval times. This new mercantile wealth not only created a new social class who incidentally were not backward in claiming the power it conferred, but also the concept of numerical calculability which has since remained an

indelible imprint and sometimes impediment within human consciousness and on human activity. Of immense importance to health
and human services was its theoretical counterpoint, namely, the
idea that a quantitatively exact interpretation of nature and human
events was possible. This idea found application as early as the 14th
and 15th centuries as is evident from the history of that time wherein statistical information about European towns and cities, particularly in Italy, is recorded. It is also without question the forerunner
of our modern system of vital statistics, which by continuing to use
morbidity and mortality statistics as its bases, in fact, then, still
measures physical health by its absence. This is a fact that almost
certainly blinds us in many ways to the real nature of health being
the interplay of mind and soul with body, and not body alone. As
city-states evolved into national states, a phenomenon that acceler-
ated to the 15th century from its beginnings in the 13th, great
emphasis was placed on the accumulation of wealth. Money in the
long term could provide the means for national expansion and the
building of empires. In the short, as well as the long and continuing
haul, it could purchase the skills and brains of those who were the
architects of the technology that drove industry and commerce
which was at the heart of the revolution we call "industrial." Cheap
labor was the grease to high profits and children were its obvious
reservoir. Without voice, without protection and without any
chance of exercising self-defense, children could be exploited with
impunity. Thus, during the 14th through 18th centuries, when
nations grew and competed for sovereignty and power over each
other, the capital on which this expansion took place and from
which empires were built was the backs and heartbreaks of children.
If they survived birth and infancy, almost as soon as they could walk
they were made to work in mines, salt works, foundries, glass works,
and all manner of industrial enterprises. While no hard data are
available, no doubt because their lives were considered expendable,
the death rates of children during these exploitative times must have
been quite horrendous. Equally so were their living conditions, if

that is what they could be called, and the ever-present sicknesses, diseases, and malnutrition that weakened them.

Yet, at about the same time, the idea that humankind was on a march toward perfection, slow though it might be, took root in human consciousness. Based on Englishman John Locke's epoch-making *ESSAY CONCERNING THE HUMAN CONDITION*, the idea that people could be liberated from the darkness of ignorance into the enlightenment of knowledge through education and the reform of social conditions and institutions took off like a brush fire throughout Europe. This phenomenon, referred to now as the Period of Enlightenment, coincided in time with the currents of agitation that led to the French Revolution. It is not surprising, therefore, that social reformers and philosophers in France became its leading exponents. The humanitarian idealism of these thinkers found its expression in the twenty-eight volumes of *Encyclopedie*, published between 1751 and 1772. Between page one of Volume One, and the last page of Volume Twenty-Eight, no aspect of the human condition, and how it could be rectified, was left unaddressed, *except for children*. The polemic within *Encyclopedie* made it clear that remediation would necessarily involve stepping on those whose interests were the accumulation of personal wealth and power, as well as the pursuit of national prestige. It was from within these tensions that the modern struggle between the status quo of exploitation, alas, still all too prevalent particularly concerning children, and the forces of social change emerged. But, a glaring omission in these noble ideas of humanitarian idealism was the scant attention given to the plight of children, which no doubt reflected the social and cultural contexts and attitudes of the times. Witness to this is attested to by the French philosopher Diderot, who had been a contributor to *Encyclopedie*. In an article entitled "Man," published circa 1790, his concern that the supply of children necessary for the forced labor necessary to the building of wealth and empire led him to declare, "*If nations and empires are interested in increasing*

their numbers they must take care to reduce the number of infant deaths."
Though clearly in default of the inherent dignity and worth of children, and very much in tune with the vested interests of the times,
nevertheless, this call to give attention to high infant mortality was
a happy contradiction of intent that led to ultimate good. In fact, for
the last century or so, infant mortality rates have been used not only
to measure the state of a nation's health, from which international
comparisons are made, but it is considered the most fundamental of
all indices presently used. Thus, through a strange twist of intent,
and by his call to apply numerical assessment of the human condition to the needs of the times, an off-shoot of the money economy
of the 13th century, Diderot of the 18th century may be said to be
one of the founding fathers of modern public health. Coincident
with this need to reduce infant mortality for mercantile reasons
were the efforts of a few brave individuals intent upon alleviating
the suffering of the children, who survived birth and infancy only to
be indentured to forced labor. Though presently reaching to all
countries of the world we presently call Western, including the U.S.
this movement began in England in the mid 18th century. In the
early 18th century, the mortality of children (from birth to aged
five) in some of London's parishes is said to have ranged between 80
and 90%. Appalled by this dreadful carnage, Thomas Coram (1668
to 1751) bestirred himself into doing something to rectify it. Being
a merchant himself, Coram belonged to the mercantile, moneyed
class. Yet, he fought and campaigned to establish a hospital for children. Such was the opposition from his confreres that he do anything that might interfere with the use and abuse of children as
cheap and expendable labor, it was not until 1741, 10 years before
his death, that he was able finally to found The Foundling Hospital
for Children in London. Although barely skimming the surface of
the problems that existed at that time, nevertheless, it was the foun-
dation of a system of hospital care for sick children from which our
present system has evolved. Out of his concern for the lack of out-
door recreational areas for children from the city slums, he pur-

chased some fields in the City of London, where now stands one of the greatest pediatric institutions in the world — The Hospital for Sick Children in Great Ormond Street. Close by are Coram's fields where to this day children exercise their limbs and lungs, a fitting tribute to one man's vision that helped to change the world for children. In 1769, Jonas Hanway (1712 to 1786) secured the passage of an Act of Parliament, making it compulsory for London parishes to send infants to the country to be nursed. He was also instrumental in organizing a campaign to protest the employment of children as chimney sweeps and in the mines. A measure of the lure of wealth at whatever cost to others, and the power of vested interests that seek the status quo, it took another 120 years before an Act of Parliament forbidding such use of children was passed in 1875. On that occasion the great humanitarian, Lord Shaftesbury, wrote in his diary, "One hundred and twenty years have elapsed since the good Jonas Hanway brought the brutal iniquity of child labor before the public; yet in many parts of England and Wales it still prevails with the full consent and knowledge of thousands of all classes." In fact, eleven years previously and in large measure the result of Charles Kingsley's novel, *The Water Babies*, a chimney sweeps act was passed limiting the employment of children; however, it had proved ineffectual due to the callous connivance of private householders, local authorities, and magistrates. Despite these apparent legalistic successes, child indenture and labor was flagrantly pursued and equally denounced. The issues came to the attention of the public in no small measure due to the serialization in the newspapers of the writings of Charles Dickens and others who described in graphic detail the searing torture that was the so-called "life" of countless children. Sadly, child labor is still a blot on the human scene. With input from countless individuals and organizations throughout the world, the staff of the International Child Labor Study Group of the United States Bureau of International Labor Affairs published in two volumes, in 1995 and 1996, comprehensive reports which define worldwide abuse of children. I think now, as then, it derives from a feudalistic attitude of mind wherein the power of might is exercised over those perceived to be powerless. Who are more powerless than children and certainly so during the 18th century when society, its pattern of living and modes of existence, were utterly changed forever by the industrial revolution? Absolutely no provision had been made to meet the social, environmental, and health needs of the people who swarmed from the dying agrarianism to the mushrooming industrial centers and cities. There was complete lack of sanitation, and infant, child, and adult death rates were astronomically high. Yet, when a few enlightened individuals raised their voices in protest against these terrible conditions, little or no attention — apart from derision — was paid because feudalistically speaking the idea of society caring for the needs of individuals was as foreign then as society not doing so is to us at this time. However, the work and writings of Johann Peter Frank of Germany (1745 to 1821), John Howard, Jeremy Bentham and Edwin Chadwick of England, F.E. Fodere of France, and Lemuel Shattuck of the United States, among others, laid the groundwork for the social and environmental reforms that eventually took place. Throughout the 19th century, the concepts they put forth — that the problems of health and disease were social phenomena of equal importance to the community as to the individual — eventually found general acceptance on the premise that healthy productivity was dependent upon a healthy workforce. Only then were measures taken to ensure clean water, safe food, and efficient sanitation together with the establishment of systems to collect statistics on humanity's vital events of birth, marriage, and death and the causes of disease and mortality. Helping to bring practical application to these awarenesses were advances journeying along other routes on the historical road map.

Significant among these were the foundations of the study of anatomy and physiology that in succeeding centuries rendered knowledge of the structure and function of the human body. Increasingly, this led to a tendency to describe disease entities based on their signs and symptoms, which itself yielded knowledge about their natural history and the circumstances surrounding their occurrence. This trend to more precise clinical observation led to the classification of diseases, thus enabling their earlier identification as well as implementation of preventive measures such as quarantine. Ironically, some of the earliest diseases to be described and classified were those that occur primarily in childhood. Parallel with these developments were the growing use of the experimental method and the numerical assessment and measurement of natural phenomena. Combined they formed the basis of the science of epidemiology, which at the dawn of the 21st century overflows into countless disciplines of human inquiry and encompasses human events from womb to tomb.

Well into the 20th century, children were not of themselves or for their own worth prime targets for the fruits of this progress, but, rather, ultimately became its unintended beneficiaries. Their center stage in the human roadmap had to await general acceptance and proof of the germ theory of disease, which didn't occur until the turn of the 20th century and the subsequent development and application of vaccines. As a measure of the time lag that occurs between knowledge gained and its application, it is interesting to note that one of the leading pediatricians of the latter half of the 19th century in the U.S. vigorously opposed the germ theory of disease. In the first edition of his book *A Treatise of the Diseases of Infants* and Children, written in 1869, several years after Pasteur's discoveries, Dr. Job Lewis Smith stated that Diphtheria, Scarlet Fever, Measles and other diseases, though dissimilar, arose *de novo* by reason of the miasms produced by decaying animal and vegetable matter. He further stated that summer diarrhea — which, in fact, was caused by contaminated and adulterated milk — was caused in the families of the poor by food given to infants as a substitute for mothers milk; the mothers absence was more than likely being due to death in childbirth or her day long work in the sweat shops and factories that exploited women at that time. In six successive editions of his book, which was the standard pediatric text in the U.S. for decades, he maintained that sewer gases and miasms were the cause of most childhood illnesses. Not until the 8th Edition published in 1896, 27 years after the first, did he concede that bacteria had a role in causation of disease, but he still held fast to his belief that their propagation depended on impurities in the air and ingesta. Meanwhile, the tremendous influx of immigrants, for the majority of whom there was inadequate or no housing, no sanitation and no running water, filth, poverty, and malnutrition was causing tremendous problems in the major cities of the U.S. — much as it had done in Europe at the outset of the Industrial Revolution. In New York City in the 1890s, 63% of all deaths occurred in children under 5 years of age and one infant in five died before their first birthday. In Boston, Chicago, and Milwaukee, 50% of all deaths in those cities occurred in children under 5years of age.[1] Far from catching the attention of the authorities, it was a small group of dedicated women who sought and fought for redress of this appalling situation. Rose Hawthorne, the daughter of Nathaniel, Julia Lathrop and others vigorously protested to any man in the Congress of the United States who would listen, that something must be done specifically for mothers and children. Over many years and with much reluctance, the Congress finally established The Children's Bureau in 1912. With a miniscule budget, its mandate was to look into the condition of children and make recommendations for corrective action. The first teething it received was money set aside specifically for health programs for mothers and children in the Shepherd Towner Act, which was signed into law in 1921 and was intended to be phased out by 1927.

Despite the noble intent of this action by the United States Congress, whose members were finally convinced of the need, it

---

[1]*Pediatrics*, (February 1998): 310.

met with hostile opposition from organized medicine. In 1922, at the spring meeting of the American Medical Association (AMA) in St. Louis, Missouri, the House of Delegates passed a resolution condemning the Shepherd Towner Act. However, on the same day, the section of Pediatrics of the AMA passed a resolution supporting the Act. By their action, the fat was well and truly in the fire and, incensed by their insensitivity to the needs of women and children, pediatricians jeered at the House of Delegates when the latter attempted to change their minds. Continued dissatisfaction in the ranks of the pediatric members of the AMA eventually resulted in them leaving that organization. In 1930, 35 of them convened a meeting in Detroit, Michigan and established a new society, The American Academy of Pediatrics, which since that time has grown in numbers and stature as an organized advocate for children. The Shepherd Towner Act lapsed in 1929 but subsequently Congress restored the program as Title V and Title VI of the Social Security Act of 1935. This provided for the establishment of Maternal and Child Health and Crippled Children's programs in each of the states. Administered by The Children's Bureau, its highly qualified and dedicated professionals created some of the finest programs for mothers and children anywhere in the world. Alas, with amendments to the Social Security Act passed in 1967, these magnificent programs were decimated and the Children's Bureau lost its focus as the guardian and promoter of programs for mothers and children. These 1967 amendments created Medicaid and Medicare, whose good intention was to provide fiscal access to medical and health care for those who could not otherwise afford it. The idea that providing access to a physician ensured comprehensive care for the varied needs of children was erroneous and one that, in its own way, the American Academy of Pediatrics and other organizations are still seeking to remedy.

Be this as it may, the needs of children have themselves changed dramatically over the past 30 years. To their remediation, we must bring new awarenesses of the roles of memory and consciousness in their causation. Memories of how children are to be regarded and treated are deeply ingrained in our collective consciousness. The contradictions of the urge to nurture them lovingly and the history of their use and abuse as possessions or chattels are a very real dilemma in the soul of adult humankind who retains power over them. Thus, despite the recent emphasis on family dynamics as central to their problems, a theme popularized by John Bradshaw in his books and television series, we still point the finger of blame at children when they rebel against the unloving use and abuse they experience in their homes — or more often, their lack of home, literally or in the real sense of that word. Either way, their profound sense of disconnectedness from love provides fertile soil for their antisocial and other destructive behaviors, including addictions.

The memories that go into surviving childhood are a part of the Collective Consciousness of humankind. We need above all to change the quality of the energies that go into its making for attempting to moderate or correct its fallout after the fact is second best and can frequently be doomed to failure. The neural pathways of infants and children are developmentally very susceptible to change. It thus becomes obvious why our attempts to change society and its present proclivity to violence must begin with children — indeed, even at or before their conception.

VIII

Children in History

The Abuse of their Souls
& the Myth and Reality Of Family
and Its Values

PEELING THE ONION of the physical causes of disease and dysfunction in children has revealed a raw wound at its center. It is the wound in the soul of who they are and how little attention has been given to its pain, suffering, and healing. It is a wound whose symptoms are being expressed in the epidemics of emotional, behavioral, and learning dysfunctions, which are engulfing children and society, and too often their feelings of powerlessness and helplessness are erupting in rage and violence.

Fortunately, we are at a point in history where the level of awareness about the soul-abuse of children is steadily rising. Yet, the memories within the collective consciousness about whom they are, how they should be treated, and expectations about their role and place in society are deeply engraved. Indeed, these memories are the building blocks upon which each generation has based its belief systems and perceptions about children, adding and subtracting to them as society has changed. We know from the abundant evidence that proves it that adult behavior is molded and in great measure derives from the quality and texture of life's experiences. It is my belief that this begins at conception. It is the memories that these experiences leave as energies within the trinity of body, mind, and soul of every individual that subsequently drive their perceptions, feelings, and behaviors. Thus, changing the energies within the collective consciousness, which dictates the belief systems of society, has a convergent trajectory with healing the injured energy of the victims of soul abuse — changing one leaves imprints on the other.

Violence against infants, children, and youth reaches us from antiquity. Willful killing of children, usually infants and usually unneeded and unwanted girls, has been responsible for more child deaths than any other single cause in history other than possibly the bubonic plaque.[1] Whipping of children and youth has been the prerogative of parents and teachers since the days of the early Greeks and Romulus and Remus. The intent was to whip them into submission; but what it actually accomplished was the perpetuation of this violence through the energy of the memories it created in its victims who, not uncommonly, developed sadomasochistic tendencies which were deposited on the bodies and souls of future generations. The extent of sexual abuse of children is reflected in the reports of Greek and Roman doctors who rarely found intact hymens in female children. The rape of little girls was so common

---

[1]Theodore Solomon, "History and Demography of Child Abuse," Pediatrics, April 1973; and Samuel X. Radbill, *A History of Child Abuse and Infanticide and Violence is the Family*, (New York: Mead and Company, 1973).

that scenes built around such incidents were a mainstay of ancient comedies and were considered to be the "funny" highlights of these stage plays. Likewise, boys were regularly handed over by their parents to neighboring men to be used for adult sexual pleasure. Indeed, Plutarch wrote a long essay on the best kind of person to choose for such activities at a time when child brothels, rent-a-boy services and sex slavery flourished. In ancient times, it was common practice for parents to hand over their children at birth to caretakers, a precursor of the nursemaid and nanny practices of later generations. However, in ancient times, it was common practice for these caretakers to abuse the children sexually and no doubt, also physically. In Colonial America, adolescents could legally be hanged for cursing or smiting their natural parents in contexts where these youths were probably rebelling against being used and abused. From their inception, schools have often been the location of violence toward youth, many employing a man in charge of the whip to punish schoolboys upon the slightest pretext.[2] This sadomasochism was undoubtedly the acting out of memories of abuse in the whipper's own childhood, a manifestation of the power of transgenerational memory and its residence in the collective consciousness. The history of children is filled with reports of nightmares, hallucinations, and terrors, as well as their convulsing fits, dancing manias, loss of hearing and speech, and confessions of intercourse with devils. The attitude of parents and caretakers toward these events was reflective of their own childhood experiences — for rather than giving comfort, they believed the best way for the children to overcome their fears and problems was to confront them head-on. They would take children to cemeteries and to gibbets from which hung the rotting corpses of those recently publicly hanged — most often for stealing to survive — and to prisons where prisoners were whipped and tortured. In hindsight, many of the

---

[2]Ibid.

afflictions these children were enduring were due to diseases such as Saint Vitus' dance and other neurological disorders.

It is a fact that historically and throughout the world parents have tended to wield absolute power over the lives of their children, even unto death if they were unwanted. The sociocultural roots of this power sprang from many sources but most particularly from beliefs inculcated by religion, concern for population control, and maintenance of a physically healthy, i.e, able to work, population.[3] The extent of parental power has led some to conclude that the history of humanity is founded on the abuse of this power as visited as abuse on children. The messages in this book and others that I have written points to my belief that this is correct. The rationale for such a stunning statement includes the fact that just as family therapists today find that child abuse often functions to hold families together as a way of solving their emotional problems, so, too, the routine assault of children has been society's most effective way of maintaining its collective homeostasis.

Just imagine homeostasis — meaning, same state — achieved through violence against children. This in itself stuns the mind and sensitivities if we have eyes and ears to see and hear what its real meaning is! But, its fallout has stunned and stunted the soul of humankind.

In the past, no matter what anxieties beset adults in their lives, children were readily at hand to relieve them through erotic beatings, incest, and torture. Yet, despite all of this there has also been a moral current, which sought to prevent or mitigate violence toward children and youth. For example, in the 16th century revulsion at the severity of punishment practiced in schools prompted Ascham to write his masterpiece *The School Master* in which he advocated

---

[3]David Bakin, *Slaughter of the Innocents: A Study of the Battered Child*, (Boston: Beacon Press, 1972).

love instead of fear in teaching children. Also, in the 17th century, the Renaissance revolt against authoritarianism influenced Comenius to advance a theory and to propose a practice of education based on the level of the child's development. More than three centuries later and within the context of the knowledge we presently have about the long-term effects of both positive and negative experiences of early life, he was quite a seer and a prophet. He asserted that teachers should conform to the developmental patterns of their pupils, a notion that alas is still not universally and fully understood or practiced, and that punishment is not an effective motivator to learning or good behavior.[4]

The attention drawn to the violence perpetuated on children in schools, factories and homes by these and several other writers, notably Charles Dickens, eventually led to social reforms, but rarely, if ever, did these reforms penetrate the fortress of the home. Undoubtedly, the prevailing dominance placed on the rights of parents and the lower public visibility of what went on behind closed doors contributed to the uninhibited and unrestricted practice of violence in the home — to the point where it was accepted as standard behavior. So great were parental rights that in 1874, in Boston, Massachusetts, when the celebrated case of Mary Ellen took place, she was removed from the appalling abuse and neglect to which she was subjected, in her home, by virtue of legislation designed to protect animals, there being no such legislation at that time to protect children. Strange and appalling as it may seem, it was legislated concern for animal welfare, combined with outrage at the unprecedented publicized anguish of one child, that eventually led to the establishment of child protection programs, whose mission today is overwhelmed by the sheer numbers of children needing their services. Yet, despite the depressing extent of child abuse today, hindsight prompts us to believe that, in fact, relations between parents

---

[4]Rolf E. Muuss, *Theories of Adolescence*, (New York: Random House, 1962).

and children have evolved through successive generations to where it may be said that, in general, parents tend to work through their own childhood traumas and anxieties in a slightly better manner when relating to their children than did their parents when relating to them. Given the facts about the present level of child abuse, this may be hard to believe, but if history is to be believed, it is so. Perhaps, as often happens, the good news gets buried under the bad, but the good news of this general trend is testimony to the visionaries of the evolution of human consciousness — particularly those who perceive it to be a circular motion of eternal energy treading a path back to its source, the Omega point of Teilhard de Chardin and the 6th Stage or Supreme Consciousness of Kenneth Wilber. Like those who have gone before us, because we are pilgrims on this journey toward *at-one-ment* with our source, it behooves us to be aware of where we are and to examine what our responsibilities are in regard to its continued refinement and redefinition.

So, where are we?

Comparisons between then and now in any context that involves family and the relationship between parents and children are subject to severe limitations due to the cultural beliefs and behaviors that historically have put up the bars to any outside intrusion. Furthermore, it is only within the last two to three decades that the reporting of suspected child abuse became mandatory for physicians and health care workers in the U.S. Even more recently, hotlines to child protection services have been established, patterns replicated in other Western countries and some, as in the U.K., predating those in the U.S. Thus, data from the reporting of child abuse and neglect are of very recent origin and, undoubtedly, still fall short of its actual occurrence. Sadly, there are still many parts of the world wherein there are *no* safeguards for children and where their use and abuse continues unabated.

Robbed of the hard data necessary for making valid comparisons between then and now, what follows is necessarily a review of the present status of the world of children — in so far as this world denies them their birthright of love, safety, and nurturance. In the U.S. in 1992, 1.5 million violent crimes were committed against children — 23% more than in 1987. Since 1988, more youth aged 15 to 19 died from gunshot wounds than from natural causes.[5] Coherently, a study conducted by the American Psychiatric Association in 1992 revealed that children witness an average of 8,000 murders and 100,000 other violent acts on television before finishing elementary school. Between 1960 and 1994, the number of working mothers increased fourfold from 6.6 million to 24.2 million, and presently 35% of children are left to care for themselves after school.[6] These societal changes have resulted in emotional overload for parents who are thus more likely to take out their fatigue and anger on their children. Despite the regularly recurring headlines of children being abused in childcare facilities, and by babysitters and other caregivers, the evidence is that those who are primarily responsible for the abuse of children are their mothers, their fathers, both parents, or their surrogates.[7]

And, yet, there is a thread that runs through the human imagination which visualizes children as safely belonging to *home* and to *family*. Yet, so often this is not the case and homelessness, along with all its attendant deprivations, is their experience. That homelessness exists at all in any society, let alone the affluent societies of the Western world, is a shocking reality. In the U.S. children and youth comprise nearly one-sixth of the homeless population that is estimated at between 2.5 and 3 million persons, and they are the fastest growing segment of it. In fact, women, children, and youth com-

---

[5]Data from U.S. Justice Department quoted in *AAP News* (August 1995).

[6]U.S. Bureau of Labor Statistics, 1996.

[7]Joseph Langa, in "Letter From the President of the American Academy of Pediatrics," *AAP News* (April 1998).

prise almost half of the homeless population, giving lie to the homeless stereotype as being an alcoholic, run-down, older, and usually white male. Horrifying as all of this is, homeless children are becoming the gruesome legacies of ethnic and religious wars throughout the world. In Rwanda alone, an estimated 3 million are homeless in addition to the 10 million who were killed.

It is hard to imagine a social environment less conducive to health and normal development than to be homeless and also a poor child, and this is the case. Differences between homeless children and children in general are large and in some cases dramatically so. The general pattern of illness among homeless children is not atypical of children's illnesses in general, but the comparative rates of occurrence frequently are inordinately elevated. The negative effects of homelessness on intellectual development and school performance are well known, as are the effects on various physical disorders both acute and chronic, the combination being now referred to as "The Homeless Child Syndrome." This comprises poverty-related health problems, immunization delays, untreated or undertreated acute and chronic illnesses, unrecognized disorders, emotional, behavioral, and other psychological disorders, school problems, child abuse and neglect, and a high incidence of alcohol and drug abuse, pregnancy, and poor nutrition.[8] Other problems include a high incidence of accidents, injuries, burns, and lead toxicity. Most homeless children of school age tend to have low scores on tests of expressive vocabulary and word decoding, and preschoolers tend to be below age expectations in receptive vocabulary, visual, and motor skills. A recent study of homeless children and their mothers in the U.S. revealed that the reasons given for homelessness included

---

[8]E. Bussuk, et al., *American Journal of Ortho-Psychiatry*, 57 (1987): 279-286; E. Bussuk and Lynn Rosenberg, "The Homeless Child Syndrome," *Pediatrics*, 85, 3, March 1990; *Today's Child*, 2,4,1988; Commission on Community Health, "Health Needs of Homeless Children and Families," *Pediatrics*, 98, 4, October 1996.

physical abuse, substance abuse, disagreements with landlords, and poor or impossible living conditions. This is replicated in other countries. One can safely assume that where there has been physical abuse, there has been verbal and emotional abuse, if not also sexual abuse and rape. The large numbers of children now on the streets and in shelters and other facilities providing services to the homeless mean that the homelessness of the 21st century is already being created today and that the lives and expectations of tens of thousands, if not millions, of children are being jeopardized and destroyed by forces over which they have no control.

The short-sightedness of a society that fails to take into account its own wellbeing by not addressing the soul distress of children was referred to by Van Doorn Ooms in a recent article which analyzed current fiscal policy in the USA. He said that by not adequately addressing the increase in child poverty, the productivity of the future labor force is threatened. For all the abuse and usage children endured in the past, they were nevertheless perceived as *immediately* essential to the money economy and the building of Empire. Nowadays, their input is more remote given laws designed to prohibit their employment until adolescence and the expectation they will be in school until aged 17 or 18, alas, an unfulfilled expectation — especially for homeless children. Remote though their future employment may appear, to a society bent on immediate profits, children are the future workforce for a workplace that will demand skills and knowledge far beyond what these disenfranchised children will be able to offer. Then, there are the throwaway kids, those who have been told to leave home or have been thrown out by their parents and the more than one million who run away each year often to escape abuse. In her book *Please Help Me God*, Sister Mary Rose McGready, President of Covenant House, America's largest shelter for homeless and runaway kids, tells the heartbreaking stories of some of these children. Entangled in a web of abuse and sex, these innocents — some as young as 10 years of age — struggle to find hope in the dark and loveless world of their knowing. But, as testimony to the love that does exist in our world, hundreds of people of all ages have dedicated themselves to helping these children and have formed Covenant House Faith Community in order to do so. Many of these volunteers live in community for 13 months and work one-on-one with the children. One has to wish that even some of the half-million youth who are incarcerated in secure facilities for major crimes such as murder had somehow found their way to one of the several locations of Covenant House and other similar resources. The inability of many children and youth to find meaning in their lives is at the root of the so-called "new" morbidities of youth: school failure; 25% of high school-students drop out of school every year; violence; and the addictions of sex, drugs, and alcohol that are in fact their cry for direction and yearning to find the meaning that is all too absent from their lives.

Visions of children belonging to the loving families and homes of their birth is further shattered by the realities of their lives lived in step-families, foster homes, and orphanages. In 1960, less than 1% of children experienced the divorce of their parents each year, but demographers now estimate that 45% of children born during the 1980s will experience the divorce of their parents before they are 18 years of age and 35% will live with a step-parent before they are 18 years old. In fact, projections indicate that by the year 2000 the stepfamily will be the most common type of American family, followed closely by single-parent households,[9] which presently is the experience of 25% of children and for a further 36%, the father is absent.[10] There is a general awareness that divorce or the death of a parent is stressful for children, but presently there is less aware-

---

[9]P. Glick, "Remarried Families, Step-Families and Step-Children," *Family Relations*, 35, 24, (1989); and Emily and John Visher, "Why Step-Families Need Your Help," *Contemporary Pediatrics* (March 1992).

[10]AAP News (August 1995).

ness that the remarriage of their parents may be even more stressful. Studies of hospitalized children indicate that the percentage who develop medical or psychiatric problems is higher among those who live with a step-parent than it is among children from single-parent households, surely giving pause to the commonly held beliefs that single-parent families are the single most common cause of psychological morbidity in children. Almost universally, children respond to the remarriage of their parents with manifestations of grief — grief at the loss of their family unit, the loss of a parent and of familiar surroundings and the loss of control over their own lives. These factors combined with conflicts of loyalty toward both parents and resentment of the step-parent inevitably lead to intense stress which is expressed in physical, emotional, and/or behavioral disorders and dysfunctions — the nature of which depends on the age and developmental level of the child and their genetic inheritance.

A similar scenario holds true for children in foster care. In the U.S. the population of children in foster care doubled in the decade 1982 to 1992 and is presently estimated to be more than half a million and continuing to rise. Despite the fact that studies suggest a higher prevalence and greater complexity of illnesses, particularly the so-called mental disorders, which are in fact soul disorders, among children in foster care, foster care programs are becoming increasingly under scrutiny for deficiencies in their management. But, in fact, they are burdened by shortages of caseworkers and availability of foster families, an over-subscribed court system and inadequate resources to track children within the foster care system itself. Agencies attempting to improve their services have to contend with the challenges of shrinking budgets, rising costs and rising demands on their resources and services. A 1994 report from the U.S. General Accounting Office (GAO) revealed that the rapidly increasing numbers of children requiring foster care is largely due to neglect resulting from the increased drug use of their parents, particularly their mothers. Ominously it also appears that there is presently a greater prevalence of physical and developmental problems in children in need of foster care due to prenatal exposure to drugs and other adverse circumstances. Even without the added burden of prenatal exposure to drugs, a child cannot develop emotionally or spiritually in a system of rotating foster homes. Yet, it has been the custom to remove a child from a foster home when bonding occurred with the foster parents lest they become too attached. The obvious absence of insight and understanding of child development that would permit and promote such inhuman policies is perilous, for with each move the child becomes less open and less able to make attachments and this rejection becomes engraved on their psyche. Concern over these issues has been ongoing for decades, and in my research I came across no less than 200 references, some dating almost a century ago. Most of this concern went unheeded, but the American Academy of Pediatrics recently codified it in recommendations for the health supervision of children in foster care.[11] Over and above these recommendations are the underlying causes for them — a sense of hopelessness in their mostly very young parents that sought connection and meaning in the fleeting moments of sex that brought an unwanted child into the world.[12] Is this what we are turning our backs on because for those with means and power it is something to read about or deal with from an unfeeling distance, as was demonstrated just a few years ago (1994) by the then newly elected Speaker of the U.S. House of Representatives,

[11]J. Goldstein, A. Freud and A, Solmit, *Beyond the Best Interests of the Child*, (New York: MacMillan, 1976); and Peter C. English, "Pediatrics and the Unwanted Child in History," *Pediatrics*, 73, 5 (May 1984).

[12]L.H. Pelton, "Foster Care Population Trends in the 20th Century," *Journal of the Society for Social Welfare*, 16 (1987): 37-62; T. Tatara, *U.S. Substitute Child Care Flow Data*, Report 9, American Public Welfare Association (August 1993); and American Academy of Pediatrics, "Health Care for Foster Children," *Pediatrics*, 79 (1987): 644-646.

Newt Gingrich? To resolve the expanding crisis of so many unwanted children, he suggested that the Government should stop all financial assistance and other benefits for teenaged and unwed mothers and use the savings to build orphanages. Needless to say, this caused quite a furious debate on both sides of the issue. In fact, it was a replay of a similar debate that took place in the late 19th and early 20th centuries as to which was the best means to ensure normal growth and development for children who were homeless and abandoned — group care homes such as orphanages or foster care parenting. Dr. Abraham Jacobi, a founding father of Pediatrics in the USA, assembled data on the fate of children placed in orphanages and in 1870 expressed his concern by saying, "The attempt to raise babies and children in great institutions, even with large means to aid you, cannot be justified. These institution must be given up and used for other purposes." At the time he expressed these opinions, most orphanages were run by religious organizations or by boards comprising wealthy women who found purpose in their lives by caring for the underprivileged; in either case, since looking after these children gave meaning to the lives of those who ran the institutions, not surprisingly his sentiments received condemnation from them. Throughout his long life he was a powerful advocate for children, and in 1889 in his address as the first Chairman of the section on Pediatrics of the American Medical Association, he spoke of the risks to infants in institutions: "The larger the institution, the surer is death. Modern civilization may be planning for the best, but being mistaken about the means it has out-heroded Herod."

Eventually, due to the general raising of awareness about the downside of orphanages, spoken to by the characters in the novels of Charles Dickens, William Faulkner, and several others, foster care became the desired substitute care for children without homes and families. Presently 75% of children in government subsidized care reside in foster homes. But, if there is a more lonely word in the English language than orphanage, we never want to hear it for it conjures up pictures of children underfed, beaten, abused, used, and living in cold and forbidding buildings often sharing beds or even sleeping in bathtubs. In a December 1994 article in *Newsweek*, Dan Dorfman, a columnist for *U.S.A. Today* and a graduate of an orphanage, said, "I favor anyplace for a child but an orphanage, it brings back bad memories to think of that place. It's a constant emotional bombing, you really don't belong to anybody, you're really in the worst kind of limbo — you don't stand for anything." Thus does he describe the soul scarring he endured and which is the experience of all children deprived of loving family and birth homes.

Alas, living in their birth homes does not guarantee children freedom from abuse and exploitation. In 1997 in the U.S. there were 969,000, i.e. almost a million, confirmed cases of child abuse, and in the same year the privately funded National Committee to Prevent Child Abuse issued an in-depth report on the problem based on 1996 figures. Significant in their findings was that children left unsupervised and uncared for by parents with drug and alcohol problems comprised the vast majority (60%) of all cases of neglect and abuse. This, of course, reflects the GAO report which stated that the increasing number of children requiring foster care is due to neglect resulting from the drug and alcohol abuse of their parents, which in turn begs attention to the hopelessness that is driving these tragedies. Neglect of this kind is invariably accompanied by physical and/or sexual abuse and, in fact, the report of the *National Committee to Prevent Child Abuse* cited physical abuse in 23% and sexual abuse in 9% of the children "reported" as abused in 1996.

Child abuse is a national and worldwide nightmare that afflicts well-to-do and middle-class families as well as the poor. Countless reports and studies attest to the high prevalence of in-the-home abuse of children of all ages and it doesn't all derive from recent legislation in the U.S. and elsewhere mandating the reporting of such occurrences. For example, in a nationwide study of 1000 adolescent girls conducted in the early 1970s, Dr. Gisela Konopka and her colleagues found an unexpectedly large number who related incidents of being treated violently by adults.[13] Twelve percent (12%) reported having been beaten, 9% said they had been raped, and 5% said an older youth or adult at some point in their lives had molested them. Significantly, Dr. Konopka had not designed her study to evaluate abuse but concluded, "Without looking for it we found the battered female adolescent." And who suffered the consequences? Not only the girls themselves but also society in terms of the illnesses and dysfunctions caused by their abuse. They spoke about feeling bad and sad, of attempting suicide and running away from the homes that harbored their abuses.

Undoubtedly, they all suffered to greater or lesser degree the soul scars that manifest as Post Traumatic Stress Disorder (P.T.S.D.), at that time not a recognized diagnosis since it is one that evolved principally from the symptoms and behaviors of the soldiers who had fought and survived the Vietnam War. The girls were a representative sample of adolescent girls of that time and came from all socioeconomic groups, from rural as well as urban areas and from a variety of racial and ethnic groups. Several who were apprehended for running away were then marched through the judicial system to a place of "correction" because of the suffering inflicted on them by others, while their tormentors were left free to dump their filth on others. Some of the girls reported being further abused in the institutions to which they were sent. What hope did these girls and countless others like them have of ever recovering from these slayings of their personhood? Sadly, little or none at all, for at that time it was the rule to blame the victim for being victimized — particularly if it was a female — a rule that is still all too prevalent today. They were left with scars that fractured their souls

---

[13]Gisela Konopka, *Young Girls: A Portrait of Adolescence*, (Englewood Cliffs, NJ: Prentice Hall, 1975); American Humane Association, *National Clearing House on Child Abuse and Neglect*, 1975; and *Children Today*, U.S. Government Printing House, 1977.

and which more than likely were passed on in some way to their children as perhaps they were passed to them from their own parents.

Likewise, an unpublished 1970 study of 200 male youths in a juvenile detention center located in Colorado found that 42% and probably more had been abused in early childhood. None of these situations had been reported either to welfare or police departments at the time of their occurrence: 38% of the youths reported having been abused by a family member within 6 months prior to the interview. Many of the youths also reported other experiences of abuse, including sexual abuse in the home, physical, emotional, and social abuse in school and foster homes, and also by police in the community. What this clearly demonstrates yet again, as if it needs to be repeated, is that children who have been abused, neglected, or abandoned are being punished for this having happened to them.

How much longer will it take for us to be fully cognizant that children do not deserve to be corrected for the absence of love and stability in their lives?

In this context our present concern with child and adolescent abuse is to be welcomed, providing we keep in mind that heretofore we have been blind to the suffering it inflicts and dismissive, if not ignorant, of the real causes of it. Connecticut Superior Court Judge Charles Gill, at the annual meeting of the American Academy of Pediatrics, in November 1996 eloquently addressed this awakening. Driven by the heartbreak of children that had been "processed" through his court and grievously wronged by adult-oriented policies, he urged members of the Academy to make an unprecedented recommendation for an amendment to the Constitution of the United States recognizing children's rights.

"I've had three children I have tried to protect in courtroom situations who on being returned to their parents were murdered by

them; it is time to stop the nation's younger citizens from being treated like pieces of property. I speak as an angry man, an angry father, an angry American and an angry judge. We are stuck in a paradigm in this country and that paradigm is that children are property, not people."[14]

The judge's perceptions were echoed in a February 1998 article in *Pediatric News* titled "The Land of Custody." It was the story of a child whose adoptive parents claimed they were unable to "control" him, even after years of prescribed drug therapy. They wished to give him away to his adoptive grandmother who encountered no problems with him, particularly when not on drugs. When the child was brought to court for a Solomonic Hearing by the Judge, the physician who cared for the child was bombarded by telephone calls from all concerned, whose intent was to persuade him to slant his report in a way that would sway the court's decision to their liking by influencing the recommendations he would make. The physician's comment was that "The land of custody will swallow you whole unless you use the only safe navigational tool there is, which is a singular focus on the welfare of the child."[15]

Horrendous as these high-profile situations are, there is that which has been so pervasive in the disciplining of children that it has until recently gone without notice. Corporal punishment and "spare the rod, spoil the child" was and remains axiomatic to child rearing. In 1950, 99% of parents said they spanked their children; 1975, 97%; and in 1985, more than 90% used corporal punishment on toddlers and more than half continued to use it into the teen years. Several studies have shown a relationship between corporal punishment and the later aggressiveness and delinquent behavior of the child. Others show a relationship between it and later emotional

---

[14]*Pediatric News*, November 1996.

[15]*Pediatric News*, February 1998.

problems such as depression and low self-esteem. Of particular interest is the consequence of harsh discipline used on girls in their tender, powerless infancy and early childhood from 0 to 3 years of age. They are more vulnerable than boys to harsh discipline and are negatively emotionally programmed by it and the accompanying lack of maternal warmth. By age 4, they have I.Q. scores on average 12 points lower than girls who receive low punishment and high warmth. Because these children are future mothers, this has special significance because what they have received is what they will likely pass on. They have been tutored probably like their own mothers before them to violence and absence of love as the resonance within their souls.

It again proves that the pivotal role of loving touch in the nurturing of children and the healing of violence in society can *not* be overestimated.

This was emphasized by research reported at a special conference on the short and long-term consequences of corporal punishment held in February 1996 and co-sponsored by the American Academy of Pediatrics and the Maternal and Child Health Bureau of the U.S. Department of Health and Human Services. Regardless of the disciplinary style of the parent, the use of positive contact with the parent was positively associated with child behavior described as friendly and outgoing.[16] Negative contact or even absent contact leads to the inner feeling of being disconnected from love which I believe is at the center of all human misery, and the soul so injured then brings about violence. The high prevalence

---

[16]"The Short and Long-term Consequences of Corporal Punishment," Supplement to *Pediatrics*, 98, 4 (October 1996); Murray A. Straus, "Spanking By Parents and Subsequent Antisocial Behavior of Children, Archives of Pediatric and Adolescent Medicine," 151 (August, 1997); and Judith Smith and Jeanne Brooks-Guinn, "Correlates and Consequences of Harsh Discipline for Young Children," *Archives of Pediatric and Adolescent Medicine*, 151 (August, 1997).

rates of corporal punishment suggest that parents have little knowledge or give little thought to its later effects. Indeed more often than not, their behavior is repeating their own experience.

It goes without saying that children need boundaries in order to grow into loving, responsible adults. They also need to learn the limits of their own testing and thereby develop respect for others. But the evidence says that replacing corporal punishment with nonviolent modes of discipline could and probably would reduce the risk of antisocial behavior in children which is so often the forerunner of adolescent and adult violence and crime. Thus, society as a whole would benefit if we ended our systems of violent child rearing, some of which goes on under the euphemism of spanking. To foster such a turnaround, the Committee on Psychosocial Aspects of Child and Family Health of the American Academy of Pediatrics recently issued its guidelines for effective discipline. Wisely, they suggested that when advising families about discipline strategies, professionals should use a comprehensive approach that includes but is not limited to consideration of the parent-child relationship, reinforcement of desired behaviors, and consequences for negative behaviors. They further stated corporal punishment is of limited effectiveness and has potentially deleterious sideeffects.

Perceiving children as chattels to be used and abused or disposed of is a worldwide phenomenon — so, too, is the mindlessness that sees them as the problem. Yet, at the same time there are glimmers of hope that we might be on the threshold of change. For example, in South Africa there is growing resentment and reaction to the large numbers of homeless children and youth roaming the streets of the large cities but one man's intervention appears to be reducing the numbers as well as the antagonism toward them. Coleridge Daniels is employed by the Salesian Institute in Capetown to work with youths, aged 15 to 24. He has gained a reputation in many sectors as a successful mediator among different interest groups. His first attempts at finding places of safety for teenagers are directed toward persuading them to return to their families, but some find the situation in their homes so unbearable they refuse to do so and in other cases parents do not want them to return. Some have spent so many years on the streets they find it difficult to change and a sizable proportion do not want to return to the circumstances that made them street kids to begin with. In other words, their connection has become the street and the other children with whom they share that life. Because they need to think of their immediate needs in order to survive, begging, stealing, or mugging for money becomes a *modus vivendi* with all of the consequences this entails. Daniels spends every morning on the streets gaining the trust of the youths who live there, and in the afternoons and often evenings as well, he runs an advice center at the Salesian Institute. Here he mediates between the youths and whomever they are in trouble with, usually the police, traffic cops, or members of the community whom they have victimized. Schools have become important to the success of the program through what Daniels describes as "positive peer role modeling." He says, "Here they get a taste of normal life and the school kids also see what it is like on the other side." Such awakenings on both sides can in the long-run lead only to greater understanding and compassion on the part of the "haves" for those who through no fault of their own have been thrown the dice of "have nots" — and, compassion is food for the soul.[17]

The world could do with several Coleridge Daniels' in all of its large cities and rural areas as well, for one-on-one is a powerful tool, as is collective people power. The latter was recently demonstrated in Belgium, a small country known for the rectitude it presents to the world as its national face. This was shattered in the summer of 1996 by a series of lurid revelations about the existence of a particularly repellant sex-torture murder ring whose victims were chil-

---

[17]Daniels, as reported in *Capetown Times* (South Africa)

dren. This, and accusations of pedophilia against top government ministers, made Belgium the epicenter of European scandal. Assessing the situation, political scientist Kris Deschouwer observed, "In Belgium we eat well, we know how to enjoy ourselves; we always knew things were wrong here but as long as we really didn't feel it, that was O.K."[18] In so saying, he touched the very essence of the problem. Feeling for self and others is of the soul; if you don't feel for others, soul is in limbo and anything goes. However, public anger and disgust at what was happening ran so high that citizen's groups organized a demonstration to demand a government clean-up and action against those who ran child sex, torture, and murder rings. Three hundred thousand people, fully 3% of Belgium's entire population, marched in the streets of Brussels calling for corrective action. For the first time in recent history it was noted, Belgians were confronting central questions about themselves, questions that in other European countries are covered by old, smug, and protective interrelationships between parties involved in such activities.

Then there are the children of war. Since 1993, the UN Human Rights Commission has worked on ending one of the worst abuses of modern times: the use of children in armed conflicts.[19] Boys and girls as young as 15 may be sent into battle without violating the almost universally accepted Convention on the Rights of the Child. In reality, many, aged 12 and younger, have taken part in fighting, mainly in Africa and Asia. The work at hand is to raise the minimum age to 18. There is, however, no consensus and when this year's effort failed in March, some felt it better to skip a year and try again in 2000. Among those opposed to setting the age limit at 18 is the U.S. which recruits boys and girls as young as 17, with parental

---

[18]*Time*, December 2, 1996.

[19]*Christian Science Monitor*, "A Responsibility to the Children," (via ClariNet), April 14, 1998.

consent. The Pentagon wants to stay with 17, as do the defense ministries of many other countries.

On the whole, the U.S. has approached the issue of children's rights gingerly. The U.S. waited years to sign the convention and hasn't yet ratified it, a position shared only with Somalia, which has no government. But there are other obstacles to agreement. Some countries like Kuwait and Cuba want no age limit on conscription in the event of invasion. And there is growing recruitment by armed groups fighting under local warlords or as part of resistance movements. Pakistan, for instance, supports Muslim fighters in Kashmir and argues that a struggle for self-determination supersedes all age restrictions.

Meanwhile, more and more children have been pressed or lured into service as soldiers or as spies, saboteurs, and transport mules. In the 40 or so armed conflicts now in progress around the globe, aid organizations estimate that 250,000 children are under arms, mostly in Africa. The UN Children's Fund (UNICEF) estimates that between 1987 and 1997, 2 million children were killed in and by fighting in wars; 4 to 5 million were disabled by war-related injuries; 12 million were left homeless by war; and that more than 1 million were orphaned or separated from their parents by war. I believe these figures are very conservative. The psychological trauma of such experience burdens the future of those involved and of the communities to which they belong. UNICEF also estimates that 6 million children in the world are starving and that 35,000 die each day from preventable causes, such as diarrhea and malnutrition.

In Romania, it was the custom under President Nicolae Ceausesau to have all orphaned children evaluated at age 3. If they did not meet expectations, they were put into warehouses of unbelievable inhumanity, tied to cots, and starved until they died.[20]

---

[20]Beverly Peberdy, "Do Robins Cough?" as in *Readers Digest* (March 1998)

Slowly but surely we are opening the curtains on the stage which is the lives of children. Disbelief and revulsion prompts us initially to close them again, for surely it must be a phantasmagoria — a delusion, a play of horrors. But, it is not! It is real! Not withstanding that, thankfully, there are children everywhere whose lives are graced with love. The question for all humanity is "What are we going to do about preventing and ameliorating further carnage on the souls of children and the adults they become?" For as the old wise adage tells us, "As the twig is bent, so grows the tree." The energies of human consciousness know no national boundaries. Therefore, as it pertains to the worth of children, it is a worldwide phenomenon that will require a worldwide will to understand that what *is* must change if we are to survive.

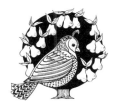

IX

The Biology of Soul

THE SCARS CAUSED BY THE MAYHEM that is the absence of love and a loving family penetrate deeply into the souls of children. Their woundedness is emotional and spiritual. It is a deeply felt sense of disconnection from their creative source which clouds perceptions of their self-worth and of their true identity as unique and irreplaceable children of Creation. This alienation denies them a vision of how they can participate with meaning in the world into which they have been born. Inevitably, this confusion and the anger it generates lead to an inability to feel respect for themselves or for others which, unless there is intervention, travels with them throughout their lives. Their consequent and frequently antisocial and violent behaviors, which in fact are cries for help and for them to be heard and taken seriously, have recently become the rallying point for politicians and others to indulge in rhetoric about "re-turning" to family values.

One presumes that what is meant by "family values" is domestic tranquillity. However, the long history of family violence and the abuse of women and children makes the domestic tranquillity whereof they speak a fantasy. Painful though it is to acknowledge, nevertheless, it is now believed that violence and abuse often served as the glue that held families together. Whereas it is now gaining public attention, in fact, it has always been there. Previously, it was rarely reported because to do so would remove the mask that protected the family name and, worse, it could open the doors to the closets wherein were hidden the secrets of shameful and dysfunctional family behaviors. For sure, the unprecedented attention currently being focused on violence might lead some to believe that it is something alarmingly new. In some ways it is, particularly as perpetrated by children on other children and adults and by the use of guns in the hands of children as young as 5, 7, and 8 years who now gun-down, murder and maim fellow students and teachers in their schools. Chillingly some of these tragedies have been executed with the precision of a military operation as happened in Jonesboro, Arkansas in March 1998. In the U.S. since 1997, there have been a disturbing number of youngsters who have fired on fellow students and teachers and in six of these incidents, multiple deaths and injuries have occurred. Sadly, some children have even turned guns on their parents and killed them.[1]

In our rush to put an end to these horrible travesties we must remember that while we can learn from the past and, indeed, *must* do so, we cannot reinvent it. In fact, given the realities beyond the fantasies of what "family" was in the past, the question is really, "How in our right minds would we ever want to?" David Ramage, Chairman of *People for the American Way*, addressed this succinctly when he said, "Many people are scared. They're being manipulated into trying to return to a world that never was and, perhaps, never

---

[1]*Time*, (June 1, 1998).

[2]David Ramage, *People of the American Way*

will be. It is a myth, a lie and a fraud."[2] And, in an other context, in his book *Priesthood Imperiled*, famed theologian Bernard Häring observed, "While nostalgia for the good old days was less dangerous in a more static era, today's yearning to turn the clock back may ultimately lead many to suffer the fate of Lot's wife and risk becoming pillars of salt.[3]

We do, of course, all of us, yearn for family integrity and domestic tranquillity. It has been there to some degree in the past, it is presently there though submerged under the welter of opposite experience and exposure, and its gifts are beyond question. Indeed, findings from the *National Longitudinal Study on Adolescent Health* show, beyond a doubt, that when there is a *felt* emotional and spiritual *connection* to a parent, parents, or teachers, adolescents are much less likely to engage in risky behaviors.[4] This finds a resonance with the fact that throughout the litany of theories about human psychology that have ebbed and flowed along with the therapies believed to effectively deal with if not heal its pathology, it has to be admitted that, for the most part, they have failed. At the root of this failure is the general inattention given to the interplay of *soul* with *mind* in the genesis of psycho-pathology, whereby the feeling part of us — the soul — becomes devitalized and its spiritual energies are deenergized. Statistics tell us that the occurrence of what is referred to as mental illness but which in fact reflects soul disharmony is on the increase. Added to the personal suffering, the cost in lost productivity in the U.S. alone is estimated at $148 billion *annually*.

Soul is not a sleeping partner in our trinity of body, mind, and soul. Indeed, it might even be that the present mayhem could

---

[3]Bernard Häring, *Priesthood Imperiled: A Critical Examination of Ministry in th Catholoc Church* (Liguori Publications), 1996.

[4]*Pediatric News*, (October 1997).

eventually be the blessing that will invite *soul* into the consciousness of a re-birthing of "family" and "family values" because it is the functions of soul expressed as feelings and the functions of mind expressed as thoughts that are at the center of society's present dysfunction. If soul is the principle of life, and the source of all life is God, and all life is encoded in memory, then soul must also operate from memory. It can therefore be perceived as that which, containing the memory of its beginning in God, seeks living union with its source in and through our response to grace. Grace, meaning gift, comes in the many faces and forms of life's experiences and in all shades of suffering and joy. But we know that the texture of our responses is woven from the fabric of our early experience beginning in or before the prenatal period. These experiences are for the most part beyond our conscious recall, as also are the memories of feelings passed to us in our genes. But, together they form the basis on which all other subsequent experience will be grafted and interpreted, and sets the stage for how immune our souls will be to the events of life that seek to disconnect us from our true heritage as children of God and of Love. How all of this plays out throughout our lives becomes a drama of continuing sequences and suspense because *soul* is always connected to the energies and promptings of its memories which resonate as our feelings, and feelings are intimately related to our thoughts, and together, they are the parents of our behavior.

For example, an infant born with genes predisposing to affective mood disorders may never fall prey to these devitalizing conditions if, immediately following birth, there is loving touch and contact with its mother and, thereafter constancy of nurturing contact with her throughout the first 6 to 12 months of life. Such contacts inject resilience and immunize against the consequences of devitalizing experiences. Denied this affirmation of loving belongingness, he or she will be subject to the expression of the negative effects of the memories that the genes carry. Scientifically, this is now premised on the knowledge that the emotional energy fields that develop between nerve cells and fibers result from the memory of the initial sensory and emotional experience.

If we tease apart the symptoms of all psychiatric disorders, their roots can be traced to a few but very powerful feelings: fear, anxiety, abandonment, sadness, and rage. Each and all of these emotions serve to disconnect *self* from original identity which results in alterations of the chemistry and energy patterns of the brain. Hitherto, we have attributed the cause of psychiatric illness to be the electrochemical changes that accompany them, believing these were inherited or simply another manifestation of the mysteriousness of disease. But, it is becoming ever more clear that electrochemical changes are responses to and the consequences of the "stressors" that change the normal energy and electro-chemical patterns of mind and body, thereby injuring both and drawing the feelings of *soul* into their dysfunction.

These changes can now be tracked and visualized with powerful new devices, which themselves employ energies of different frequencies to map those operating in the brain. Positron Emission Tomography (PET) tracks blood flow, considered a proxy for brain activity, as does Single Photon Computerized Tomography (SPECT). Superconducting Quantum Interference (SQID) picks up magnetic fields as a sign of brain action and Magnetic Resonance Imaging (MRI) snaps detailed images of the brain. Research using these technologies has rendered intriguing information, not only of how the brain functions, but the differences in male and female responses when presented with the same challenges. For example, researchers have reported that men and women use different clumps of neurons when they take a first step toward reading and when their brains are idling: the female response being more embracive.[5]

---

[5]*Newsweek* (April 20, 1992); and *Time* (July 17, 1995).

Other researchers have mapped brain activity during hearing, speaking, seeing, and thinking. Opening a window on brain activity leads one to concur with the comment made by Dr. Crick, co-discoverer of the structure of DNA, that the brain is the most complex entity so far "discovered" in the universe. Powerful imagery though this may be, I believe it will pale in the yet to be discovered interchanges and vortices of energies that maintain life functionally, whose disruptions and interruptions result in disease or dysfunction and whose common origin throughout all time is the changes in memories brought about by adaptation to the many causes and forms of *stress*.

Regardless its quality, there are no barriers to the circulation of energy throughout body, mind and soul, and therefore the effects of *stress* are not limited to one or the other, but permeate all three. Stress may be defined as an imbalance between environmental demands and the coping resources of the individual or, simply stated, an imbalance between the inner and outer worlds. In general, this mismatch or lack of balance manifests in three major ways: first, by causing changes in the normal physiological functions of the body which, if unrelieved, then leads to physical disease — it is estimated that between 85 to 90% of all illness is stress induced, second, subjectively, by causing thoughts and feelings of distress; and, third, behaviorally, in disturbed personal and interpersonal functioning and performance.

The reaction to stress derives from one of the oldest memories that we carry within us; the physiological response which we call the "Fight" or "Flight" reaction. In the latter part of the 19th century, Claude Bernard, the great French physiologist, pointed out that the internal environment of living organisms must remain within fairly constant physiological and, thus, functional parameters despite changes in the external environment. Otherwise, dysfunction and death will ensue. The coordinated physiological processes, which maintain this internal stability or homeostasis, are achieved in two ways: first, by a very specific reaction to the stressor that is provoking the imbalance; for example, the shivering and cold extremities we experience when exposed to low temperatures, both of which combine to diminish loss of heat from the body, second, by a non-specific reaction of total internal readjustment. Dr. Hans Selye, who pioneered the medical research on stress, showed that this non-specific response calls forth the same biochemical, hormonal, and nervous system changes regardless the nature of the original stressor, be that physical, chemical, or emotional or, as is usual, a combination of all three.[6]

He called this The *General Adaptation Syndrome*, a process of internal readjustment directed toward rebalancing the body's functions and systems and acting independently of the specific stressors that caused it. We call the changes that bring about this readjustment, *The Stress Response*.

The observable and measurable signs of the stress response are increased heart rate, breathing, blood pressure, metabolism, and muscle blood flow. But, what happens at the functional and energy levels of the body during the stress response is very complex. There is a release of chemicals, hormones, and neurotransmitters from the brain which sets in motion further hormonal and metabolic changes. The adrenal glands release their chemicals and neurotransmitters, including adrenaline, cortisone, and related steroids, which cause active release of glycogen from the liver resulting in a rise in blood sugar. This increase in blood sugar, and the surge of adrenaline plus other factors, readies the body for fight or flight which was the original purpose of the stress response. In days gone by when men and women lived closer to nature, and food had to be hunted, the fight or flight reaction was a very necessary protective mechanism. If a bear was on your tail, you would need that surge of

[6]Hans Selye, *Stress Without Distress*. (Signet: New York, 1975).

adrenaline and blood sugar, a fast heart rate, and rapid breathing to propel yourself up the nearest tree. But in today's society, when we are under stress, there is usually no place where we can run to. In common parlance, "All stressed up with nowhere to go!" We are caught, as it were, with all that energy and chemistry churning inside of us with no viable outlet — the reason, of course, why exercise is so good for us at any time, but particularly in times of stress. In order to sustain this reaction, the demands of the body for amino acids, vitamins, elements, and other nutrients increases. If we factor into this equation the denaturation of our foods, the need to supplement the diets of those in stress, children and adults alike, with appropriate doses of vitamins becomes apparent.

In addition, and *central* to the ultimate fallout from stress, which manifests as disease or dysfunction, is its effect on the Autonomic Nervous System. There are two major components to the nervous system:

1. The *Somato-Sensory*: which controls movement, sensation and speech and, so long as we remain healthy, is more or less under voluntary control

2. The *Autonomic Nervous System*: which controls all other body functions

In essence, it is the steward of every organ and system in the body. However, the autonomic nervous system itself responds, interplays with, and is controlled by the hypothalamus and the limbic system and, through many other connections, interfaces and communicates with all other parts of our being and with our many layered consciousness.

The control buttons for the autonomic nervous system are located in the hypothalamus which then in a sense may be regarded as a fuse box for the body's electrochemical and other messenger systems, all of which operate on memories of how to react once given a signal specific to a particular situation. These in turn are relayed to and then respond to messages from the limbic system, the oldest part of the brain, which controls emotions and from the cerebral cortex where thoughts are processed. The hypothalamus communicates with the endocrine system through its connections with the pituitary gland and, through special neural connections, communicates with the entire immune system which during stress slows down its functions: T-cells diminish and have a slower rate of DNA repair, immune globulins are diminished, cortisol is increased and other interferences with normal immune functions occur.

Dr. Hans Selye described three stages of *The General Adaptation Syndrome*: The first stage he called the stage of "The Alarm-Reaction;" the second stage he called "The Stage of Resistance" or "Adaptation;" and, the third stage he called "Exhaustion" or "Burnout."

Stage One is, for the most part, good. The alarm rings, we are warned, and if all goes well and we deal effectively with the stressors, the body rebalances itself and returns to normal. If the stress is maintained over a period of time without relief, the body begins to fail in its normal balancing process and the cascade of events that I have outlined takes on a more permanent character. The body actually adapts to the stressors and attains a level of functioning above and beyond its optimal level.

Stage Two is when *stress* becomes *distress* leading to pervasive dysfunctions which if unrelieved can become permanent. The hypothalamic connections I have just described impact on consciousness — and therefore on thought and perception. When thought and perception become compromised, we begin to see the world as through a darkened mirror. Our moods and our behavior become dysfunctional, and since we as children of God are spiritual beings on a human journey, therefore more than body, mind, and emotion, when these are off-balance it creates a sense of disconnectedness from our spiritual core which manifests as spiritual devitalization.

Stage Three is when the body is overwhelmed and death ensues.

As mentioned previously, it is estimated that between 85 and 90% of all illness is stress induced. From what I have described, quite clearly the process of disease and dysfunction originates in Stage Two of the General Adaptation Syndrome or, as we also refer to it, the stress response. The determining factor of which type of disease will ensue is genetically determined and is a function of the memories within our own unique genome. This factor, which at present is not in the universal awareness and thus little if ever discussed, is vital in the delicate balance that exists between health and disease. The reason for its importance is, I believe, that fundamentally it is a replay between what is within and what is without. In this case it is the tension(s) that exist at the interface where health and disease tumble together and mix with the two major energies: that which is within — deriving in part from our genes and in part from the memories encoded in our response systems from past experiences — and that which is without — which is our present reactions to circumstances and environment. When this combination is juxtaposed with the interchangeable nature of matter and energy, and the changeability of energy itself, it takes on profound importance in terms not only of its role in the genesis of disease but also in terms of its prevention and treatment.[7]

This scenario takes on even deeper meaning when applied to the stressors and the stresses that weaken the soul and which set the stage for psychiatric disorders. The consequences of stress that result from injury to the soul have for too long been submerged under the overabundant attention given to the physical conse-

---

[7]For further reference, see U.M. Anderson, *Psalms of Children: Their Songs and Laments*, (She Bear Publishers: Ellicottville, New York), Chapter 4, pp. 61-77.

quences of stress. But, within the context of child development, which is the matrix of whom we become as adults, it takes on enormous importance because when there is early onset of soul stress and distress, original identity becomes damaged to the point where dysfunction resulting from the changes in memories and energy ensues, allowing violence to take root within the soil of its despair.

As with the stress response, it may be said that in general there are three stages of reaction to soul trauma which are identifiable from early infancy onward. In the first stage, there is confusion. Hence, several competing emotions struggle for expression. Basically, it is a reaction of grief at the trashing or invasion of personhood or of its neglect and abandonment. The resulting sense of powerlessness and helplessness lead to denial, sadness, anger, and even blind rage. In infants and young children, this leads to the syndrome called "Failure to Thrive." The child withdraws from its unloving and often hostile environment, refuses to eat, shrinks from touch, and, if there is no intervention, will die. During and following World War II, many infants and children were orphaned and put in orphanages where they were simply warehoused. Death from the absence of love was a frequent occurrence.[8] In recent years, events and wars all over the world have inflicted similar horrors on these innocents to the tune of the death of millions of them. Those who survive the early onset of soul trauma invariably exhibit in later childhood signs of Reactive Attachment Disorder of Infancy and Early Childhood (RADIEC), whose symptoms act like tentacles squeezing and inhibiting the energies within the soul.[9] The suffering of these children, those who survive as well as those who don't, cry to the world for the nurturance of the sacredness of their beings.

---

[8]John Bowlby. *Child Care And the Growth Of Love*. Abridged and edited by Margery Fry (1953). Based on permission of the World Health Organization on the report *Maternal Care and Mental Health*.

The second stage of soul trauma is a period of transition wherein the emotional effects of the trauma become grafted onto the personality of the individual. It can last from several months to a year or more depending upon the age of onset and how well immunized the soul had been prior to the attack on its integrity. By this, I mean how well ingrained are the memories of connectedness to love and creation. This, of course, depends on the quality of the energy from the beginning of life as well as on the energy in the genes and the environment within which the child subsequently exists. The more positive these energies, the greater will be the resilience and, therefore, also the resistance to permanent dysfunction. This is why the energy of parents during and following conception is so vital to the well-being of their children. But, for children who have endured the early onset of soul trauma, the dysfunctional behaviors classified as adjustment disorders of emotion and behavior which characterize this second stage and which appear from about the age of two on upward — combined with the long-term sequelae of RADIEC —

---

[9]*Reactive Attachment Disorder of Infancy or Early Childhood* (RADIEC): (A) Markedly disturbed social relatedness in most contexts, beginning before the age of five, as evidenced by either [1] or [2]: [1]-persistent failure to initiate or respond to most social interactions (e.g., in infants, absence of visual tracking and reciprocal play, lack of vocal imitation or playfulness, apathy, little or no spontaneity; at later ages, lack of or little curiosity and social interest); [2]-indiscriminate sociability, e.g., excessive familiarity with relative strangers or making requests and displaying affection. (B) The disturbance in A is not a symptom of either Mental Retardation or a Pervasive Developmental Disorder, such as Autistic Disorder. (C) Grossly pathogenic care, as evidenced by at least one of the following: [1]-persistent disregard of the child's basic emotional needs for comfort, stimulation, and affection. Examples: overly harsh punishment by caregiver; consistent neglect by caregiver; [2]-persistent disregard of the child's basic physical needs, including nutrition, adequate housing, and protection from physical danger and assault (including sexual abuse); [3]-repeated change of primary caregiver so that stable attachments are not possible, e.g., frequent changes in foster parents. (D) There is a presumption that the care described in C is responsible for the disturbed behavior in A; this presumption is warranted in the disturbance in A began following the pathogenic care in C. Taken from DSM-III-R (313.89).

take on more ominous long-term prognoses than those who have not.

The third stage is one of consolidation. The trauma takes up a felt residence in the soul whose message is that all that is external to personhood is hostile and to be feared. This fear expresses its disconnection from the source of love and creation in serious psychiatric disorders and in violence inflicted upon others and often upon self. These psychiatric disorders are classified in the *Diagnostic and Statistical Manual* of the American Psychiatric Association (DSM-IV) according to their symptomatology, but they all derive from the same source — soul trauma — whether the symptoms fall into the category of affective disorders, the many so-called personality disorders, or the complex assortment of dissociative disorders such as schizophrenia, multiple personality, manic-depressive disorders, and others.

The type of disorder is determined genetically. This means that at some point in the lives of our familial ancestors, they reacted to soul stress in a way that stressed the capacity of particular genes that control emotions and behavior to maintain balance and function. If these weakened genes and *their altered energy* find no surcease from their vulnerability and fragility in succeeding generations or are assaulted by further trauma, they will continue to manifest as soul dysfunction and psychiatric disorder, all depending on a critical level of environmental stress that will release their dysfunctional energy in Stage Two of the General Adaptation Syndrome in those who carry them.

It is, I believe, altered energy and its altered messages that initiate and then maintain the electrochemical changes in body and brain which being measurable have up until now been believed to be the cause of psychiatric disorder. If this is so, then the implications for treatment and healing take on an unprecedented aura of light and hope. For by changing the quality of the energy, we change the quality of life's experience.

Thus, it is clear that to inflict trauma on the soul, whether it be one's own soul or that of another — worst of all a child's soul — is to darken the light of love and weaken the bonds of connectedness to its source in God. To be separated from source by whatever means is surely a property and dimension of evil.

This is often poignantly brought to my attention when a child who has been removed from its parental home because of neglect or abuse will ask me, *"When can I go home?"* What they yearn for is to be and to feel connected and the only connectedness they have known is their experiences in the "family" home. And yet, when you ask them what they most yearn for, invariably they will tell you love, which speaks eloquently to the power of the energy of the drive to *love* and be loved that resides within the memory of our primal source regardless our human experience. No matter how blurred it may be, it is always there. Furthermore, if we know that it is the memories and their energies within the genes that govern their function and that these memories and energies can be altered by experiences both personal and transgenerational, then our biology is and has been fashioned at some level and at some point in time by the quality of the energy within the experiences that created the memories. Surely, this is a major interface between nature and nurture and one that gives us hope because it implies that the restoration of functional memories in the genes of the individual, and in the Collective Consciousness, can be accomplished by effecting changes in the quality of the energy that drives them. This also engages our concepts concerning Free Will and the expectations we have of it, particularly in situations where we believe that applying it will change destructive behavior.

Free will implies the ability to choose. But, if our biology is to a large extent a "given" from which our behavior derives, then this must either enhance or diminish our ability to choose. Asking some-one to exercise "will power" in situations requiring positive choices to be made when the givens militate against such a possibility, only deepens the imprint of these memories when failure ensues. Rollo May said it well when he stated, "... In a contest between Will and Imagination, Imagination will always win."[10] Has anyone caught imagination on a screen or is it a word we use to describe the ener-gy that drives us? I believe time will prove the latter. In the April 1998 issue of *The Atlantic Monthly*, Edward Wilson wrote an inter-esting article on this topic entitled "The Biological Basis of Morality." He asked, "Do we invent our moral absolutes in order to make society workable or are these enduring principles expressed to us by some transcendent or God-like authority?" He went on to respond by saying that "while efforts to resolve this conundrum have perplexed and often inflamed the best minds for centuries, it appears that the natural sciences are telling us more and more about the choices we make and our reasons for making them."[11] He observed that each kind of animal is guided through its life cycle by unique and often elaborate sets of instructional algorithms, there-fore, it seems reasonable to assume that human behavior originated in the same way. It is my belief that at the center of these algorithms is the *energy* within the memories transmitted genetically and the changes that have occurred within them from generation to gener-ation and that in many parameters they are species-specific. Although imprinting of one species on another does take place post-natally, nevertheless, it appears that species-specific memories, together with the primal memory of creation and love, are never lost. But, in terms of transforming dysfunctional behavior, resulting from the biological "givens" that themselves have resulted from

[10]Rollo May. *Love and Will* (W.W. Norton and Co: New York), 1969.

[11]Edward Wilson, "The Biological Basis of Morality," *The Atlantic Monthly*, (August, 1998).

alterations over time and from personal experience, restoration of functional behavior will depend on restoration of the functional memories and energies from which the genes and other carriers of energy operate. All of this gives us much food for thought and reflection on the paradigms we presently use to solve our human dilemmas. For example, we constantly are told that the best way to counter the causes of crime is to create better schools and neighborhoods where young people can learn nonviolent routes to social status. The "War on Poverty" of the 1960s poured billions of dollars into such programs and the statistics concerning violence and crime have quadrupled since then, informing us that not only was this a failure, but that such pursuits lead to dead-ends. Aggressive promotion and marketing of drugs by the pharmaceutical companies that manufacture and make billions of dollars of profit from them, combined with the Western pursuit of instant answers for every problem have led to the commonly held but fallacious belief that there is a drug to cure or control every disease or dysfunction. Drugs can *never* cure or fix anything. At best, they enable the body to heal itself. The dangers of their over use and abuse cannot be too strongly stated. Indeed, it is now the common endeavor of pediatricians and other healthcare professionals to re-educate parents about the dangers inherent in the indiscriminate use of antibiotics for conditions where they are not indicated. This follows on three generations of parents who demanded antibiotics for their children at the slightest hint of a sneeze or a cough. Now, pediatricians worry that, when truly indicated in severe infections, the bacteria may have learned how to become resilient to them, a situation that is becoming of deep concern. Of course, what we are dealing with is changes in the memories of attack learned by numerous strains of bacteria when repetitively confronted with bacteriostatic or bacteriocidal antibiotics. With their lessons well learned, they have literally changed the rules of engagement and the game plan itself. Lessons from this experience need now to be applied to the use of psychotropic drugs.

Currently, it is quite a common occurrence for parents and teachers to ask for, if not demand, psychotropic drugs for a child at the slightest hint of nonconformity, inattention, or inability to fit into a classroom routine. On several occasions I, myself, have been handed a note from a teacher by the parent or surrogate accompanying the child to my office, which bluntly states, "Give him/her Ritalin!" There is no question that we are experiencing an epidemic of attentional and behavioral problems among children, but drugs will not ease this dilemma either for the child, the family, or society. The chemical imbalances that lead to dysfunction are the result of assaults emanating from many sources on the normal development of the brain and its neural pathways. The ultimate and only solution is to address these causes and to remove or downsize them. In this regard, we should take a lesson from the microorganisms that have learned to outwit their nemesis, which was antibiotics. Engaged as we are in reeducating parents and child-care givers about the dangers inherent in the indiscriminate use of antibiotics, now we should be adding warnings about the possible long-term sequelae of the indiscriminate use of psychotropic drugs. Their effects in the short and longterm on the developing brain and neural pathways are not known. It is within the realm of possibility that changes in the energy interfaces of adults who received psychotropic drugs as children will be or already have been passed on to future generations, altering permanently modes of function and behavior; such a scenario casts a dark shadow over the future and calls for letting go of the paradigm of a drug for every problem. It likewise overshadows the majesty of human biology and threatens its future unfoldment by deepening the fear to look at biology and its forebears as central to the human condition.

For example, a Harvard geneticist warned in 1984 that if human social organization is a direct consequence of our biologies, then nothing short of some gigantic program of genetic engineering could possibly make significant alterations in social structure. Well, *if* genes were merely unalterable matter, fixed as it were in concrete, he would be right. But, this is not the case. Their memories and the functions they control are frozen or consolidated energy and,

energy can be changed.

Given that this is so, there can be nothing inherently, let alone permanently, deterministic about biology or a biological perspective. On the contrary, when placed within the winds and changes of the energies that control all life, the expectation for biological change makes perfect sense. While biology shapes our impulses and aptitudes, it does not act alone. It functions within the context of personal experience and the energies within the person's environment — physical, emotional, and spiritual. This is really great and good news and explains why even though genes susceptible to various negative conditions are inherited, i.e., are biological givens, they may never cause disease if the early bonding experience and environment of the individual militates against this occurring by the dominant presence of positive and nurturing energies. This concept is already begetting a whole new approach to the prevention of cancer in women known to carry susceptible genes for breast and ovarian cancer. In this instance, one hopes that modalities involving positive energies will be more universally employed and added to the positive visualization and other methods pioneered by the Drs. Simonton some years ago.

Harvard researcher Dr. Mary Carlson recently reported that orphaned children deprived of maternal attention had abnormally high levels of cortisol. Cortisol is a powerful hormone that plays a major role in the body's response to stress. The greater the stress and the inability to cope with it, the higher the levels become. Her comment was interesting: "This clearly shows that there are physiologic consequences to sensory deprivation along with the behavioral abnormalities we all know about." One wants to add an "AMEN!" by saying, "Of course, because given the interdependence of body, mind and soul, you cannot have one without the other." It is time for us to not only know but to apply what we know to the alleviation of behavioral dysfunction. It is not something that just happens. It is always the consequence of the altered physiology that in turn results from the changes that occur in the energy patterns of the brain and nervous system which in turn again are due to changes that have occurred in the memories of healthy functioning. These are triggered primarily by the absence of *loving touch* at or immediately following birth, as well as by inadequate or absent maternal affection and attention before and immediately following birth. These are situations that society, given the will to do so, can address and redress. It adds scientific and measurable testimony to the observations of the late, great Dr. Erik Erikson who perceived emotional problems to be the consequences of arrested development. If we put his observations into the context of the arrested flow of energy leading to interruption in the flow of one developmental level to the next, then it adds a whole new view on how we should be addressing release of this damned-up energy so as to allow healthy development to continue.

In the July 1997 issue of *Vaccine Bulletin*, there was an article that called for reducing "missed opportunities" to immunize children against the physical diseases of childhood.[12] When we immunize against these diseases, what we are really doing is changing the memories and energies in the child's immune system that will serve to protect them against the consequences of attack by the organisms that cause the diseases. Note it does *not* protect against attack, but only against deadly or debilitating consequences. This exhortation comes at a time when immunization levels are the highest ever recorded and the killing fields of children and, therefore, of society are emotional, behavioral, and soul disorders. Is it not now time for us to turn our attention to reducing "missed opportunities" to

---

[12]*Vaccine Bulletin* (July 1997).

immunize children against the debilitating or deadly consequences of the interruptions to the flow of nurturing energies that result in diseases of the soul? As adoptive parents have discovered, giving love is sometimes not enough for a child whose early imprinting was deprivation and abuse. Sadly, this is too often the case in children adopted from overseas orphanages, which is presently a concern of the American Academy of Pediatrics (AAP) Committee on Early Childhood, Adoption and Dependent Care, whose intention is to help adoptive parents before as well as after the fact.

Given what we know about the pivotal role that memory and consciousness play in human perception and behavior, and the forces to which they bend, laudable as these and other efforts may be, nevertheless, fundamental and lasting change requires that we seriously focus our efforts on the beginnings of life. The energies present at conception, during pregnancy, and immediately following birth are probably the greatest influences on the quality and texture of our entire lives. They are the nutrients of the soil in which the soul takes root and grows. It flourishes if the soil is tended with love and the energy of connection that flows through the channel of being wanted, all of which becomes the infrastructure of its functional biology and giving to it strong resilience to withstand life's testings. If the soil is needy for these nutrients or devoid of them, the soul will experience a lifetime of being in need of nurturance, which, if given, may help it in fits and starts and hopefully may help to heal it, but if absent will lead to its death. If from the start there has been negative energy to whatever degree, its memory and the damaged biology that ensues from it will remain despite whatever may be done later to correct it, making resilience to life's experiences less spontaneous. In these situations, resilience will be in direct proportion to the quality of the energy in which the soul dwells at times of testing. This latter renders further emphasis to what has already been said about the desirability of reexamining the nature of free will, and explains why current approaches and modalities used in remedial programs whose number is legion and thirst for funds unquenchable so often fall short of expectations.

Surely, the biology of the soul should lead us out from under the weight of the paradigms we presently carry and into new awarenesses of how we may immunize the soul against all that seeks to injure and diminish it.

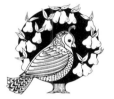

X

The Paradigm for the Future

WE USE THE WORD "PARADIGM," as I have used it in this text, to convey the form and structure of belief systems. By so doing we somewhat obscure the majesty of its full and original meaning. In the story that is the myth of Er, Plato uses the word paradeigma to mean the cloak that covers and accompanies individual destiny. One could say that this is, in fact, the energy that emerges from creation and travels as a constant companion on a unique frequency with every human being. In his book The Soul's Code, James Hillman retells the belief of Plato and his later disciples, the neo-Platonists, that each soul is given this paradeigma before it is born in human form and that it holds the pattern that should be lived by that soul while on earth.[1] He points out that

---

[1]James Hillman, *The Soul's Code*, (Bantam Books: New York, 1997).

in the last passage of the myth of Er, Plato tells us that by preserving this belief we may better preserve ourselves and thus prosper. In other words, the myth has a redemptive psychological function and a paradigm of psychology derived from it can inspire, guide, and comfort a life that is founded on it, which in the ultimate serves to give meaning to its inevitable suffering. Co-habitating with each unique destiny is the memory of its creation in divine love, which is a shared heritage of all humankind. Within this frame rests the portrait of every child entering the world through the portal of collective consciousness, but, also, carrying the gifts of their own unique identity and destiny that has the potential to influence and change this collective energy and memory for the better.

But, what have we done and what do we do to the wondrous gifts they have to offer?

The history of children informs us that there has been little awareness and even less concession made to their gifts of *soul* and *paradeigma*. Even with the most noble of intentions, the tendency has been and continues to be to bend them to the expectations of the adults in their lives. Even if they escape the extremes of abuse, misuse, and neglect, they endure many pressures to conform to parental and societal values. These tensions may, indeed, be a part of their soul's learning and journey, but they are also the source of much intergenerational conflict, conflicts that are almost always arbitrated by the exercise of adult authority and control over the child. And, what does this do to the child? At best, attempting to mold them to the energies alien to their *paradeigma* leaves them in a limbo of identity, which causes anxiety and confusion. At worst, the rage and rebellion at being victimized and not being heard frequently finds its outlet in antisocial acting-out and self-destructive and addictive pursuits. However, until we accept as a given, and put into our consciousness what we know about the power of memory and consciousness in human perception and behavior, our attempts to heal their negatives will fail until we grant children their fundamental and essential role in the becoming of humankind to *at-one-ment* with God. While this, of course, means ensuring their physical integrity and well being, of equal importance is providing the means for their spiritual and emotional nourishment and integrity. Fundamental to this nourishment is adult respect for their unique soul and *paradeigma* and the treasure of primal love they carry within them which, alas, too often becomes a silent partner throughout their life span. In his masterpiece *The Prophet*, Kahlil Gibran speaks eloquently to this scenario. When the woman who was holding a child to her breast asked the prophet, "Tell us about our children," he replied:

> *Your children are not your children.*
> *They are the sons and daughters of Life's longing for itself.*
> *They come through you but not from you,*
> *And though they are with you yet they belong not to you.*

> *You may give them your love but not your thoughts,*
> *For they have their own thoughts.*
> *You may house their bodies but not their souls,*
> *For their souls dwell in the house of tomorrow,*
> *which you cannot visit, not even in your dreams.*
> *You may strive to be like them, but seek not to make them like you.*
> *For life goes not backward nor tarries with yesterday.*

> *You are the bows from which your children as living arrows are sent forth.*
> *The archer sees the mark upon the path of the infinite,*
> *and He bends you with His might that His arrow may go swift and far.*
> *Let your bending in the archer's hand be for gladness;*
> *For even as He loves the arrow that flies,*
> *so He loves also the bow that is stable.*[2]

---

[2]Kahlil Gibran, *The Prophet*, (Alfred A. Knopf: New York, 1968), p. 17-18.

The imagery is beautiful and the "bow that is stable" speaks to the strength of parenthood that allows the child the freedom to fly. But, they too were once children and they bring to parenting the memories of how they were parented and the energies that were present throughout their own development.

Dr. Erik Erikson, who died in May 1990 at the age of 92, was in our time one of the great seers of human development. His observations and his work remain a highly influential model of the human life cycle, a mosaic in which body, mind, and soul merge in the dynamic process of forming an individual's identity. As a young man in Vienna, while training to become a psychoanalyst, he experienced a moment of self-doubt. His talents were in the visual arts, particularly cutting images into wood. "How," he asked Anna Freud, "could an artist help people as a psychoanalyst, a technique that alas requires abstract theorizing and verbal skills?" Anna put the question to her father. "Tell him," said Sigmund Freud, "that perhaps he might teach others how to see."[3] This he eventually did by elucidating the psychosocial crises appropriate to each of the eight developmental stages that he perceived as consisting the entire human lifecycle, from infancy to old age. He described his eight stages in terms of their healthy and unhealthy outcomes as follows:

STAGES OF DEVELOPMENT

I.   TRUST VERSUS MISTRUST

Approximate Ages — Birth to 18 Months

Positive Outcome: Infant develops attachment to primary caretaker and trusts that the environment regulates and responds to his/her needs.

[3]*America*, August 13, 1994.

Negative Outcome: Environment is not responsive to infant's basic needs and primary caretaker is either absent or abusive, resulting in feelings of rage and helplessness as well as fear of abandonment, possibly leading to a psychopathic life.

II.   AUTONOMY VERSUS SHAME AND DOUBT

Approximate Ages — 18 Months to 3 Years

Positive Outcomes: Parents encourage child as she/he exercises her/his autonomy, resulting in enhancement of self-esteem and confidence as well as development and self-reliance.

Negative Outcome: Parents are overcontrolling and do not allow child to express autonomy, and child internalizes feelings of shame, doubt and disapproval, possibly leading to being scared of letting people down – obsessive/compulsive behavior and paranoia.

III.   INITIATIVE VERSUS GUILT

Approximate Ages —3 Years to 6 Years

Positive Outcome: Child admires and emulates adult role models and pursues goals with a sense of purpose.

Negative Outcome: Child develops punitive conscience, which paralyzes his/her efforts due to fear of punishment, possibly leading to guilt and sexual dysfunction.

IV.   INDUSTRY VERSUS INFERIORITY

Approximate Ages – 6 Years to 12 Years

Positive Outcome: Child develops awareness of special skills and talents and engages in goal-oriented behavior.

Negative Outcome: Child realizes that she/he is inadequate in comparison to peers, a sense of inferiority develops, and child refrains from possible learning experiences, possibly leading to anxiety, depression and/or conduct disorders.

V.   IDENTITY VERSUS ROLE CONFUSION

Approximate Age — Adolescence — Moral Structure beginning to coalesce.

Positive Outcome: Person forges identity and determines which occupational role best utilizes his/her unique abilities.

Negative Outcome: Person is paralyzed by the inability to make decisions regarding career and experiences helplessness and confusion as a result, possibly leading to mid-life crises.

VI.   INTIMACY VERSUS ISOLATION

Approximate Age — Early Adulthood

Positive Outcome: Person commits to intimate relationships and is willing to make the necessary sacrifices such an affiliation demands.

Negative Outcome: Person avoids intimacy, preferring to isolate the self and becomes self-absorbed and self-indulgent, possibly leading to perceiving people as objects to be used and personality disorders.

VII.   GENERATIVITY VERSUS STAGNATION

Approximate Age — Middle Adulthood

Positive Outcome: Adult is concerned with enriching the future generation and with preserving and passing on her/his collected knowledge and experience.

Negative Outcome: Adult is unable to direct future generation due to lack of meaning or purpose in own life, possibly leading to violence.

VIII. EGO INTEGRITY VERSUS DESPAIR

Approximate Age — Late Adulthood

Positive Outcome: Adult views life as worthwhile and meaningful and accepts death as the inevitable end.

Negative Outcome: Adult experiences profound sense of despair with the realization that there is limited time remaining and he/she has not accomplished what was hoped for.

Believing, as he did, that moving healthfully from one stage to the next depended on how well the individual had resolved their earlier crises, he was in tune with nature's pattern of orderly progression from one step to the next in development and attainment of each and every skill. For example, a child's ability to walk is preceded by the ability to stand on two legs, which in turn is preceded by crawling, sitting up, rolling over, and holding it's head erect. Each of these milestones along the road to ambulation has its expected time of attainment. If there is delay at any point, it will have a domino and delaying effect on subsequent stages, the final outcome depending on the cause and degree of its severity. This is a rule that pervades the territories of every aspect of human development.

In recent years, it has become a popularly held belief, bordering on dogma, that the first 3 years of life are the most important in establishing life-long healthy psychosocial as well as physical development. Important though they are, their role is eclipsed by the energies that preside over conception, prenatal life, and the birthing process. It is self-evident that all development begins at conception, and the feeling part of us, the soul, is no exception. Therefore, while Erikson's brilliant research and insights in human psychosocial development hold validity and serve as valuable guideposts, they beg knowledge of the texture and quality of the soil from which they themselves derive. Therefore, attention focused on the role that post-birth experiences play in the genesis of emotional and behavioral disorders, while being laudable, will always fall short of giving clues and, therefore, the tools for their correction and/or prevention until and unless we include the memories and consciousness that were the matrices from which they grew. These memories are conveyed through various energy systems of which the most talked about currently are genes.

Genes are power houses of memory, each having a specific duty of form and function, which are passed from generation to generation as are their memories of how to interact with other genes so that the whole becomes greater than the sum of its parts. They are the perfect example of the interdependence of matter and energy: their residence at particular locations on their chromosomes never changes and is the same for all, but they perform their duties by means of energy over many frequencies. It is a scenario comparable to a radio station — grounded and immovable, but from where a great number of different messages can be transmitted over a variety of different radio wave frequencies to locations both near and far. The quality of the sound will depend not only on the integrity, quality, and strength of the transmitter and receiver, and the environments within which they are located, but also the environment and atmosphere through which the messages must travel. When the quality of the sound received is poor, we say there is interference. So also it is with genes. The quality of their energies, and their ability to interact with the energies of other genes, are modified by the environments in which they operate.

From womb to tomb, the environment is in a state of constant change, which no doubt explains at least in part why identical twins sharing identical genes do not behave identically nor do their genes. For example, if an identical twin is schizophrenic, the sibling with the identical gene, which when stressed leads to schizophrenia, has only a 50% chance of having the disease. Indubitably this is because the environmental experiences of each twin have called forth different responses and, therefore, different energy interactions, in the one case allowing the gene to kick in the electrochemical and other energy changes that manifest as schizophrenia and in the other case preventing it. The message is clear. What is within the genes is not always fixed and the quality and frequencies of the energies within their memories are subject to change, a phenomenon we refer to as mutation, which hitherto has been cloaked if not in mystery itself, then in one of its close relations. Since energy is flexible not only in terms of its own kin, but in its relationship with matter, mutation must work both ways, i.e., from functional to dysfunctional form and function and vice versa.

In this regard, recent research suggests that the close relationship between the negative effects of the stress response and the penetrance of genetic memories begin *in utero*. This lends profound insights into the genesis of many aspects of human feeling and behavior and is proof that it leads to prebirth bending of the intended identity of the developing individual and a dimming of the primal memory of its loving and creative origin. Over time, the permutations of these interactions have altered the memories and energies in the genes and, thus, their original messages. These mutations reside in the collective consciousness making us as a race no longer able to clearly see ourselves as children of creation, which was our original identity. Instead, fear has taken over and overtaken us so that we now perceive ourselves as combatants in a never-ending war of one-upmanship and enmity with the other.

This flawed inner ecology flows without interruption into the rape of outer ecology, and its origins are well documented in two recent studies. One sought to determine if multifaceted interventions *following* the birth of low-birth-weight infants decreased the incidence of the syndrome known as, "Failure to Thrive." The results showed conclusively that it did not. This study was the best of all possible designs and so it is almost impossible to seriously question its findings. It was conducted as a collaborative study in eight large university hospitals throughout the U.S. and was a prospective study involving 914 infants born prematurely. The interventions consisted of weekly home visits during the first year of life and bi-weekly thereafter until the age of 3 to provide in-home family support. These visits were also used to implement two curricula and ensure attendance at a child development center from 1 to 3 years of age, 5 days a week, whose purpose was to deliver an early childhood intervention. The incidence of failure to thrive did not differ between the treatment and control groups — 20 vs. 22%. Furthermore, there were no differences between the two groups in any of the outcome variables; these included those pertaining to growth, health, behavior, and three-year intelligence quotients (IQ). Interestingly, however, after controlling for multiple independent variables, significant differences in the 3-year IQ were noted in children of families that were most compliant with the interventions. The findings of this study point not only to the immediate consequences of intrauterine stress resulting in preterm delivery, but to its long-term effects and the quantitative differences deriving from the degree of parental involvement. It seems reasonable to assume that parents and families who were more compliant with the interventions were more motivated and, therefore, more accepting of the child both pre and postnatally, which means that these children were proportionally less stressed than those whose families were less compliant.[4]

Another study, whose objective was to determine which factors from the early developmental histories of maltreated children are associated with the signs and symptoms of Post-Traumatic Stress

---

[4]P.H. Casey, K.J. Kelleher et al., "A Multi-faceted Intervention for Infants with Failure to Thrive: A Perspective Study." *Archives of Pediatric and Adolescent Medicine* 148 (October 1994).

Disorder (PTSD), came to conclusions that serve to underscore the nightmare of stress that some infants, particularly those who are unwanted, endure during their intrauterine lives. The negative fall-out on soul development can only be described as soul destroying. From their findings, the authors concluded that PTSD may be caused by factors that are discernible in the first year of life and which leave a maltreated child vulnerable to this disorder. *Such factors, they said, may depend on genetics and/or events that occurred during pregnancy.* The factors they cite are not only compatible with dysfunction of the autonomic nervous system (ANS) that occurs during the stress response and Stage 2 of the General Adaptation Syndrome, but also symptomatic of it. Pervading all systems, they include suppression of immune system functions and increased susceptibility to infections, vomiting, diarrhea, sleep problems, frequent crying, fussiness, jumpiness, and distress when touched or moved, the latter reflecting not only dysfunction of the ANS, but the memory of un-loving touch. All these symptoms and behaviors reflect profound fear and anxiety, and all are observable from immediately following birth.[5]

The constant companions of our human journey, be it long or short, are the energies in our consciousness deriving from the memories we inherit from our ancestors and the memories of our intrauterine and birthing experiences. Therefore, a child born with evidence of having experienced the distress of stress prenatally and/or in the first months of post-natal life is already primed to dysfunction of its feeling soul, as well as to physical disorders. Conversely, the energy systems of infants who have not endured this assault on their beings are set to function responsively. Does the insight this gives to us harbor the secret of the origins of that great gift and staying power we call *resilience?* And, is it also the reason

---

5Richard Familano and Terence Fenton, "Early Developmental History and Pediatric Post-Traumatic Stress Disorder." Archives of Pediatric and Adolescent Medicine 148 (October 1994).

why some can engage their destiny within the mosaic of the human drama and the suffering this often entails while others cannot? *Herein is the nucleus of a new paradigm in our understanding of the fundamentals underlying child development, human behavior, and the genesis of violence.*

If we put it into the context of the evolution of human consciousness, it points unequivocally to how the primal memories of our origin in creation have become dimmed and of how our original identity has become blurred and sometimes twisted. In many places along the lineage of our common inheritance, and through all manner of God denying man-made and natural disasters, the distress of stress has changed the energies within our memories, most often to assist survival, but sometimes with results incompatible with the fullness of life. A simile is the parlor game of "Pass the Whisper." By the time it reaches the last recipient, only a fraction resembles the original message.

If *paradeigma* means the role that each soul as expression of universal spirit chooses or is given for its human journey prior to its incarnation, then in the light of the stress and distress that many infants and young children endure both pre and postnatally, particularly those who are unwanted, one has to ask to what end and for what purpose is the script and the model defaced? It seems inconceivable that a soul would voluntarily choose a life whose energies would be damaged to the point that it was constantly at war with its intended unfoldment and fulfillment. Perhaps, then, defacement of the model was unintended and, if so, have these dichotomies evolved from the mayhem we refer to as evil and is this the real as well as the mythic meaning of *Hell*, the place to which Lucifer and his minions are said to have been banished after the failure of their struggle to wrest power from the God of Creation?

The Judeo-Christian scriptures tell us that in their continuing battle for supremacy over God and Good, these fallen angels prowl the earth seeking whom they may devour. Indeed, this is brought to the attention of all who nightly pray the psalms of the prayer of Compline wherein the writer warns against these predations and the wiles of the predators. While one can glimmer the psychology of a numbers game, nevertheless, these struggles and the archetypes involved in battle are certainly a part of the collective consciousness of humanity and, when expressed within the individual, becomes a personal hell. In situations where there has not been excessive stress experienced during a soul's intrauterine life, could the transgenerational memories of ancestral stress explain why early promise and hoped for achievement forever lie fallow in some individuals? If so, it suggests that injury to *paradeigma* occurs transgenerationally, which echoes in the affirmative to that perennial question, "Are the sins of the parents visited on their children?" Sin, in this context, is synonymous with stress and the concessions energy made to it at some point along development. If so, then it is easy to conceptualize how addictions and all behavior destructive of self and others are the consequences of the struggle to be in touch with primal memory when one is stuck in the morass that has been left in the wake of its theft. Ultimately, this leads into an understanding of how violence and crime entered into our knowing and of the forces that keep them a part of the human scene.

Within this context it has been said of many who exhibit antisocial behavior or who are stuck in their addictions that they know not what bedevils them or how they can become unglued from their devilish behavior. What overwhelms them is often interpreted as stubborn refusal to change. But, when there has been no intervention in the early onset of the stress response, the electrochemical interactions of body, mind, and soul have been set at a dysfunctional behavioral level — rather like having a car engine engaging high gear and going nowhere because the brakes are locked. So it is true, they do not know what bedevils them because the discomfort of dysfunction is the energy that is familiar to them

Because so many children are unwanted and have experienced stress *in utero*, this dysfunction has become their life sentence and explains why it is also frequently observed these days that a generation of child and adolescent predators has taken over the world. An example is the story of Brian. His adoptive parents returned him to the agency from which they adopted him because they feared for their lives. He was an arsonist and very violent. Another is 10-year-old Eric, who threatened his adoptive parents and other children. He killed animals by pounding them to death and asked Santa Claus to give him a gun. Like Brian, he was unwanted and in foster care before he was adopted. Although he showed no overt emotion about his brutal ways, he was scared of his feelings and actually prayed to God for them to change. There are countless other such children in the world and, in a terrible sense, they are doing to others what was done to them, and yes, even before they were named.

One day I overheard two 7-year-old boys talking with each other in the waiting room outside my office.

"What are you here for?" one asked the other.

"I killed a cat," he replied.

"Oh, yeah. How (*note: not "why"*) did you do that?"

"I banged his head on the wall."

"Oh, that's illegal," said the other.

"Yeah," said the killer.

After a pause, the other asked, "What was his name?"

"Don't know," replied the killer, "and who cares. Trouble is, I got caught."

The only glimpse of feeling in this entire conversation was when the confidante asked the killer the name of the cat. Yet, he himself revealed that the behavior was related to legality rather than feeling. And, as the killer revealed, for those whose souls cannot feel, being caught in crime is the only issue. It is innocence lost whose awful legacy is the absence of responsibility for one's behavior.

Always evident to a greater or lesser degree in children and adults with emotional and behavioral disorders, it begets a culture wherein the evil it spurns is perceived as outside of *self* and, therefore, ultimately, no one is to blame for anything. To some degree, this is true because *paradeigma*, both individually and collectively, has at some point in development and over time been injured; therefore, blame can be placed on *other* rather than on self. But, blame is the futile exercise of using the past to excuse the inadequacies of the present. And, by perceiving what is in negative terms, it is the denial of hope that change is possible. But, if we are to embrace the unfolding of human consciousness, our task now is to use the past to understand the present and, with the knowledge gained, to create a new paradigm for the future. In the odyssey that is the *Immunology of the Soul*, we have traveled to the ports of call on whose soil the wars that begat the wounds began and have encountered some of the terrible suffering they have caused. *Now!* is the time to enter the havens wherein reside the possibilities for healing and the release of *paradeigma* to shed its creative light upon the earth.

It will take root when we commit ourselves to immunizing children, and the adults they become, against the diseases and dysfunctions that dim the light and obscure the majesty of the soul's intended destiny. Though we live in a society that seeks a quick fix for everything, exploration of the ports of call we have visited in this odyssey leaves no doubt that who we are and who we become begins its flow in the timelessness of existence and before we are conceived. Changing the landscape of these territories will not easily yield to quick fixes, but rather to the reseeding and cultivation of their soils over time.

This will begin when we teach children from a very early age about the sacredness of life and its procreation, which begs for parenting in all of its dimensions: emotional, psychological, spiritual, and developmental, as well as physical, to be an integral part of every school curriculum. In this regard, many children have told me how much they yearn for their beginnings to have been different, and they were not referring to the first 3 years of their lives, which is currently the focus of popular attention. They *were* talking about the circumstances of their conception and their experiences while in the womb. They have taught me and, indeed, confirmed the abundant evidence quoted and referred to throughout this edition, that the memory of the quality of the energy surrounding conception remains with us *forever* — as do the memories of our sojourn in the womb, as well as those during and following birth.

Included in these memories are the technological and other intrusions of prenatal care. We must question and diligently seek answers to the possible long-term deleterious effects of routine and costly procedures, such as ultrasonograms. Research has shown that in the short-term, they do nothing to improve the immediate outcome of pregnancy. *However, it is not beyond the realm of possibility that they may be interfering with the normal development of the central nervous system and, if so, may be contributing in no small measure to the current epidemic of attentional disorders and other behavioral problems.*

Similarly, the Glucola test for pregnancy-induced diabetes, administered at 28 weeks of gestation could be setting the electrochemical software of the unborn child to the memory of its rush – planting the seed of an unconscious hankering for similar rushes during its independent life. This could possibly lead to the early onset of drug and alcohol abuse, particularly in times of stress, the first step, perhaps, toward addiction. Data on the value of this test, in terms of the number of mothers identified with pregnancy-induced diabetes, are hard to find but urgently needed. Meanwhile, other tests that would diagnose maternal diabetes without affecting the unborn child should be substituted since the Glucola test could be creating long-term physical and behavioral problems for the child.

Bonding of infants to both parents, not only immediately following birth, but throughout the prenatal period should be an integral part of pre-natal care and requires more, much more, than teaching Lamaze techniques. Instructions about parenting in all of its dimensions and the use of light, color, and music to create inner calm and peace should be taught, preferably by women with this knowledge and a sensitivity for delivering and teaching it. Learning and applying such skills have obvious life-long benefits that serve to enhance personal welfare and, by overflow, thereby enriching family life as well.

In light of the overwhelming and incontrovertable evidence of the detrimental effects environmental pollution is having on the developing bodies, minds, and souls of children all over the world, we must be tireless in our efforts to become a part of the conscience of those who manufacture these poisons. Surely, given the will for change, we can find ways to use technology to clean up the mess that presently exists. It has been done before in the U.K. and the U.S.A. and it can be done again. Included in environmental toxins is the pornography and violence that saturates the media, the internet, and the so-called video games known to just about every child. Current emphasis on deescalating such readily available violence must be vigorously pursued. Why, one must ask, cannot similar talents be applied to portraying images of human nobility and the power of good over evil.

But, for the children who presently, and for the foreseeable future, need help to deal with their personal and family dilemmas –

What are the pathways along which they can be led to their resolution?

Very simply, by teaching them how to monitor and regulate the energies of their own emotional and behavioral responses to the stresses of life. There are several modalities of self-regulation that share the same hoped for and intended outcome namely, the conversion of self-defeating beliefs and behaviors resulting from hurtful memories and experiences into desired and life enhancing physical, psychological, and emotional responses.

From earliest times, and at the heart of all religious practices of East and West, self-regulation has been and continues to be sought, through prayer, meditation, and contemplation. The earlier that prayer becomes a part of a child's life, the more indelible will be its beneficial memories of connection to God and the source of creation, therefore, the more reflexive its use throughout life. Hitherto, meditation and contemplation have been considered adult pursuits, but recent reports of the tremendous benefits following classroom instruction and use of meditation in young children prompt the suggestion that it should be more universally taught and practiced.

While hoping that these time-honored ways of self-realization will become a part of every child's life, sooner rather than later, there are several ways, more secular in nature, that may be more readily acceptable. Breath, and the control of breath, is their shared entrance into the kingdom of the soul, and deep breathing is its doorway. Of itself, deep breathing allows the body to flow into the relaxation response whose physiological benefits enable optimal functioning of the autonomic nervous system and, thus, of the human trinity of body, mind, and soul. Brain activity is slowed, allowing its electrical rhythm to move from the rapid (ß) beta rhythm of involved activity to the slower (α) alpha rhythm of focus and calm. This clasps the mind and its thoughts, which then fasten to the feelings of the soul. While in alpha rhythm, the chemistry of neurotransmission changes making it impossible to feel anger or to respond in a hurtful or violent way toward other. Research also indicates that alpha accelerates learning, improves memory, and enhances creativity. Surely these benefits and the simple way in which they can be engaged invites the inclusion of deep breathing as a daily part of school activities. For children aged seven and older, deep breathing accompanied by the silent repetition of previously chosen positive affirmations or mantras is often all that is required to engage the positive energies and benefits of the *relaxation response*. As they mature and wish to move into more sophisticated ways of self-regulation, auto suggestions of balance, based on Emil Coué's methods, and many other techniques of systematic bodily relaxation pioneered a century ago by Dr. J. H. Shulz, may be added; these latter require someone to speak the instructions or, alternatively, they can be administered by way of tape recordings.

Imagery and visualization, which invoke imagination, are widely used for teaching adults self-regulation. Despite the fact that overcoming resistance due to the real experiences of life can, at first, prove to be an obstacle, it is generally very successful. Children are naturals for such therapy because they live in a world wherein imagination overtakes reality. Play and the toys that accompany it, story telling, miming, play-acting, and more, are journeys into their fertile imaginations from which flow images of what the world could be or even as they wish it to be. Using imagery and visualization, children learn self-regulation much faster than do adults and the lessons so learned stay with them longer.

Countless studies report how children have been successfully trained to turn around undesirable habits, moderate anxiety, and the many symptoms associated with chronic diseases and pain. In addition, controlled studies have documented the abilities of children to self-regulate peripheral temperature, transcutaneous oxygen, brain stem auditory evoked potentials, and many other physiological and patho-physiological processes. Most recently it has been shown they can self-regulate certain immune responses.[6] This and other research leaves no doubt that early training of children in self-regulation provides important preventive and therapeutic interventions for them, thus leading to an enhanced quality of life for them and for society. For children who are emotionally and behaviorally dysfunctional, it could prove to be their salvation.

All of this begs the question that if early training in self-regulation can provide therapeutic and preventive interventions for the emotional and behavioral disorders that lead to dysfunction and violence, why are we not doing this for all children now? It should become as much a part of the school curriculum as the three "R's." Time should be allotted to its practice on an equal basis with sports. To give it a name for the curriculum, I suggest *cyber biology*, in the Greek meaning, "that which steers, the helmsman," and in the Latin, "to govern." Cyber biology is then the art of the ability to self-regulate. In its teaching and practice, modalities must be matched to the developmental levels of the child.

Over the many years of my practice, I have developed simple ways of accomplishing all of this. In our preliminary encounters, in addition to allowing them to tell the stories of their life's experiences in their own words, I ask them among other things to tell me about their favorite and least favorite colors, sights, sounds, people, and places. I ask them to attach feelings to each of these items. Then, I begin by teaching them how to breathe deeply and rythmi-

---

[6] Wayne Rusin. "Relaxation Methods and Children With A Range of Illnesses," *Pediatric News* (November, 1988); see also, L. Kuttner, *American Journal of Clinical Hypnosis* 3, 30-34, 1988 and *Pediatric Annals*, March, 1991; and K. Olness and G. Gardner, *Hypnosis & Hypnotherapy With Children* (Grune & Stratton, 1988); Mark Smith, "Biofeedback," *Pediatric Annals* (March, 1991); William C. Wester, Donald J. O'Grady, *Clinical Hypnosis With Children* (Brunner Mazel: New York, 1991).

cally. This puts them into a state of deep relaxation, during which I do some cleansing visualization with them — guiding them to their favorite place which interestingly and most often features flowing or falling water. I use those surroundings to create a calm and peaceful energy within them. I then have them circulate that beautiful, powerful energy around their bodies and when they feel it everywhere in their bodies, I ask them to raise the first finger of their right hand. I am able to confirm their readiness by the colour in their cheeks because deep relaxation enables the autonomic nervous system to function at its optimum, one of the results being improved circulation. Next, I ask them to think of someone or something that they love and to scan their body and point to the place where they feel those warm and happy feelings the most. Not surprisingly, they most often point to their hearts, sometimes to their heads. Following this, I ask them to give those feelings a colour which is usually a soft pastel blue or pink and sometimes yellow. Then, with deep breathing, I have them circulate that colour throughout their body until they feel it pulsing everywhere. I next ask them to think about what causes them anger and to show me where they feel it. Again, not surprisingly, they point to the solar plexus, a major relay station for the autonomic nervous system whose functions are major casualties of the stress resulting from emotional dysfunction. Again, I ask them for a colour. With boys it is most often red and with girls, black. These colour choices are interesting because red is the colour of the root *chakra* whose energies interact with the sexual organs and what is the most usual crime of angry and powerless men? It is *rape*. So we know that the frequencies of anger in men correspond to the frequencies of the root *chakra*.[7] This is powerful knowledge! With girls, anger leads to depression and in the absence of colour, they see black. Again, this is very interesting because it reflects the

---

[7]Chakra's are the dynamic centers through which energy is distributed as it enters and exists the body. There are said to be 13 such centers, 6 minor and 7 major of which latter, 6 interrelate with the endocrine system.

absence of light and colour in their lives. When you juxtapose the two, it reveals that the creative power of the feminine is crushed by the abuse that leads to anger; whereas, in the male, it is transformed into an act of savagery. Do we need to look further for the bedrock of violence?

Having located the place where the anger is felt the most, we do some visual surgery. We remove the lump of anger by scooping it out and replacing it with the happy feelings and colors we had previously circulated. As they remain relaxed, I point out that it was they, themselves, not I, who accomplished all of this and that with practice they can learn to be in control of their feelings and their lives. Before they leave, they choose a stone and a piece of velvet cloth from the collection I keep in my office of the colour and texture they identified with happy feelings. I ask them to feel the stone and the cloth and to imagine that colour and texture circulating throughout their body. The reason for this is that the neural pathways of touch are very powerful and release energies according to the nature of the stimulus: loving touch nurtures; violent touch destroys. I tell them to keep the stone and cloth in their pocket and when the urge to react negatively overtakes them, to touch and rub the stone and cloth and let the memory of the good feelings they initially generated take over.

Most children need practice for this to become an instinctive reaction; therefore, practice time should be arranged, especially for children with emotional and behavioral problems. Taping therapy sessions for future and daily use, while being an obvious way to enhance these skills, is not always a realistic option. The children most in need of therapy are initially too distracted and unfocused to independently follow through on using them. However, adding biofeedback to children developmentally able to use it and interpret it adds a further dimension of empowerment for them. Indeed, research has demonstrated that children take pride in being able to demonstrate, via biofeedback, their control over various physiologic responses. Their families are similarly benefited as are also their school peers and teachers when they learn the rewards of personal responsibility through the simple application and practice of self-regulatory techniques. From the age of eight, I believe combining relaxation methods with biofeedback should be a weekly part of the school curriculum.

There are, of course, other ways of bringing about these physiological and subjective changes, some with an emphasis on changing energy from negative to positive overtones. Latterly, some of these modalities have been subsumed under the title "Re-Birthing," a reference to the biblical injunction that unless a person be born again of the Spirit he or she will not have life.[8] The energies within children are in constant flux. Accessing them and then directively changing and grounding them usually presents little difficulty to therapists who have been trained to do this. Changing the quality of energy — re-birthing — is a powerful therapy for children who bear the burden of negative energies surrounding their conception, intrauterine, and perinatal experiences — likewise, for those who suffer from Reactive Attachment Disorder of Infancy and Early Childhood (RADIEC). Yet, because we live in a society expectant of quick fixes, dependence on drugs to "fix" children is sadly all too pervasive. Although there are instances where drugs may be indicated and even helpful, in the vast majority of cases they are *not* the answer. Indeed, giving drugs to children is a still-to-be-told tale of possibly terrible burdens on their immature and still developing nervous systems and neural pathways. Indeed, in the future we may learn that the use of psychotropic drugs may have added to their problems. In this regard, we should learn from the consequences of the overuse of antibiotics, which has resulted in their diminished

---

[8]John 3: 3-8.

effectiveness and the emergence of resistant strains of microorganisms. The many faces of the scars on the soul are the expressions of memories of disconnection from our source — which no drug can permanently heal.

From all that has been said and explained, it is apparent that only by changing the energy of negative memories and thus their expression in consciousness by using self-regulatory techniques can long-lasting benefits ever be accomplished. Juxtaposing what is possible and relatively easy to do for children in this regard, which for the most part, is not being done, particularly for those most in need of soul healing *vis-à-vis* their otherwise usually well-covered physical management begs the question — *why? Why not?* What is the impediment? In the ultimate, as well as along the way it begs a radical rethinking of whom we are and how we come to be as children of eternal memory and the ever-becoming of our shared consciousness. This will require not only the *will* to change our out-worn concepts, but the *imagination* to foresee the blessings of doing so. In the immediate, there is no impediment because we don't need the huge expenditures of money — belief in whose magic so often in the past betrayed our expectations.

The *all* that is needed is the same passionate commitment, politically and socially, that hitherto has called forth the best in humankind for the benefit of all. If we put our hands to this plough, we can re-seed memories and consciousness, and accomplish for the present killing fields of humankind what we accomplished so magnificently and efficiently for those of the past.

Our thrilling tale of exploration has come to its close. No doubt, you the reader, have kept Joshua, our protagonist, in mind and have related some of what you have read, to him, and are wondering how his particular story ended.

Alas it must be said that the knowledge and awarenesses of the inner science that have been explored in this book were not there for him, (and millions others like him), at the crucial times when their application would have resulted in successful intervention in his cycle of despair. For a while he did well. He participated in visualization and at times was so pleased with what he accomplished in terms of wholesome feelings, he would smile and say; "Oh Man, that feels good!"

I also used therapeutic touch with soft toys and the special gift of a puppy, to which he became very attached.

But one day, unable to resist the taunting of a bully, and the mean look on the bully's face, he lost control and punched and injured his tormentor. His life long experience of injury, hurt and disconnectedness sewn deeply into the memory banks of his soul, and the beliefs they confirmed in his mind, took over. As a consequence, charges of assault were filed against him. During his appearance in court, his demeanor and body language left no doubt that he knew what the outcome would be, for they shouted for all to see, of his inner despair and his power-less-ness to change the cruel circumstances of his life.

Ironically punishment was meted to him for his human reaction to circumstances he had no part in creating. The judge sent him to a secure institution some distance away, from which he later escaped. From then on I lost contact with him, yet in my mind and soul there is little doubt, that being homeless and full of rage, he would turn to crime to survive, if not also to get even. And then, if he was lucky enough to survive in the jungles of street life, the wages of crime would eventually imprison his soul and its vehicle, his body, perhaps for-ever in this life.

ADDITIONAL READING:

U.M. Anderson, *Using Light and Color in the Management of Learning and Bhavioral Disorders in Children, and as a Means to Reduce Violence.* Paper presented at "Light '98", International conference, Reading University, Reading, UK., July 1998.

Jack Scwarz, Human Energy Systems. (E.P. Dutton: NY), 1980.

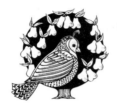

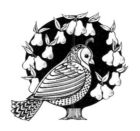

Epilogue

"The Soul makes headway solely by the Light that God has given her, that being her own, presented to her by God as a bridal gift. God comes in love with the intent the soul may arise that she may be energized above herself. Soul does not initiate the work of grace – (*sic*: since that is not her nature, and grace is a gift of God) – *till she is gotten yonder where God is plying Himself where the work is as noble as the worker* — *his own nature in fact."*

— Meister Eckhart

G OD'S INTENT THAT THE SOUL may arise and be *energized* above herself and become one with God's own nature has throughout the ages been bent and twisted. And now the human soul mourns its loss and cries to be immunized against all that assails it. The task is simple and, yet, the means to accomplish it are formidable, but no more so than was the task of finding means to immunize against the physical diseases that formerly decimated humankind.

Soul's energy accompanies all else that is passed to us from our parents and then is captive to the energies it subsequently encounters. Therefore, immunizing the soul demands that children must be wanted from the moment of their conception and, thereafter, nourished with the many energies of love throughout their sojourns in the wombs of their mothers, the birthing process, and the first hours, days, and months of their lives. Absence of this love creates the stress of disconnection from their creative source, leading not only to soul distress and a dimming of its light and power, but also to the disordered physiology of the Stress Response. This sets the buttons of genetic electrochemical and energy interchanges of body, mind and soul, at dysfunctional levels. If unrelieved, these dysfunctions accompany the individual throughout their life span and then are passed from generation to generation. They manifest as the personal hells of physical, emotional, and behavioral disorders and the fear and hatred that begets wars within families, between families, and between ethnic and religious groups and nations.

Hitherto, we have sought the causes of these many afflictions in the variables, such as poverty, that are frequently associated with them. But, it is clear that memory and consciousness and the energies that drive them are at the root of whom we are and whom we become. Such knowledge invites, if not demands, that we release old belief systems and allow new paradigms to be fostered in the genesis and understanding of all human dysfunction and suffering and, in particular, of soul (psychiatric) disorders and, in the ultimate, of violence itself. Likewise, it invites new paradigms of our approach to their healing and prevention, which will be the promise, spoken of by Meister Eckhart, of the release of soul into its true nature as one with God. A promise foretold in the Hebrew Scriptures, by the prophet Habakkuk, who pleaded:[1]

---

[1]Habakkuk 1:2-3; 2:2-4

How long, O Lord? I cry for help
> but you do not listen!
I cry out to you, "Violence!"
> but you do not intervene.
Why do you let me see ruin;
> why must I look at misery?
Destruction and violence are before me;
> there is strife, and clamorous discord.
Then the Lord answered me and said:
> Write down the vision
Clearly upon the tablets,
> so that you can read it readily.
For the vision still has its time, …

And, the time is now !

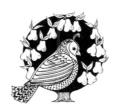

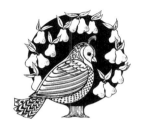

Appendix

TABLE 1

Immunization	1992	July–Sept, 1993+
DTP/DT*		
3+ doses	83.0 (80.8, 85.2)	89.9 (86.9, 93.0)
4+ doses	59.0 (56.1, 61.9)	74.8 (69.9, 79.7)
Polio		
3+ doses	72.4 (70.1, 74.7)	80.4 (75.8, 84.9)
Hib**		
3+ doses	28.2 (25.6, 30.9)	60.3 (55.0, 65.7)
Measles	82.5 (80.2, 84.8)	85.9 (82.0, 89.8)
Hep B		
3+ doses	—	15.7 (12.1, 19.2)
3DPT:3polio: 1MMR	68.7 (66.2, 71.2)	78.7 (74.2, 83.2)
4DTP:3polio: 1MMR	55.3 (52.5, 58.1)	71.6 (66.7, 76.4)

+ Provisional data based on Quarter 3
* Diphtheria-tetanus-pertussis/diphtheria-tetanus. ** *Haemophilus influenzae* type b

NOTE: Data are based on household interviews of a sample of the civilian non-institution-alized population. Refusals and unknowns were excluded. Percentages in parenthesis indicate 95% confidence intervals.

SOURCE: National Health Interview Survey: National Center for Health Statistics and National Immunization Program, CDC (Centers for Disease Control).

TABLE 2

Infectious Disease	Critical proportion of the populationto be immunized for eradication%
Malaria(*P. falciparum in a hyperendemic region*)	99%
Measles	90 - 95%
Whooping Cough(*pertussis*)	90 - 95%
Fifths disease (*human parvovirus infection*)	90 - 95%
Chicken Pox	85 - 90%
Mumps	85 - 90%
Rubella	82 - 87%
Poliomyelitis	82 - 87%
Diphtheria	82 - 87%
Scarlet Fever	82 - 87%
Small Pox	82 - 87%

SOURCE: National Health Interview Survey: National Center for Health Statistics and National Immunization Program, CDC (Centers for Disease Control).

TABLE 3

Kindergarten/1st Grade Immunization Status   %
1980 – 1993, United States

Year	Measles	Rubella	Mumps	Polio (3+)	DTP (3+)
1978/79	93	91	83	92	92
1979/80	94	93	86	93	94
1980/81	96	96	92	95	96
1981/82	97	97	95	96	96
1982/83	97	97	96	97	96
1983/84	98	98	97	97	97
1984/85	98	98	97	97	97
1985/86	97	97	96	96	96
1986/87	97	97	97	97	97
1987/88	98	98	98	97	97
1988/89	98	98	98	97	97
1989/90	98	98	98	97	97
1990/91	98	98	98	97	97
1991/92	98	98	98	97	96
1992/93*	98	98	98	96	95

Provisional data as of March 14, 1994.

SOURCE: Centers for Disease Control.

TABLE 4

Recommended Childhood Immunization Schedule January – December 1998, U.S.

*Vaccines are listed under the routinely recommended ages. **Bars** indicate range of acceptable ages for immunization. Catch-up immunization. Should be done during any visit when feasible. **Ovals** indicate vaccines to be assessed and given if necessary during the early adolescent visit.*

Age → Vaccine ▼	Birth	1 mo	2 mos	4 mos	6 mo	12 mos	15 mos	18 mos	4-6 yrs	11-12 yrs	14-16 yrs
Hepatitis B	Hep B-1	Hep B-2			Hep B-3					Hep B	
Diphtheria Tetanus Pertussis			DTaP or DTP	DTaP or DTP	DTaP or DTP			DTaP or DTP	DTaP or DTP	Td	Td
H. influenzae Type b			Hib	Hib	Hib	Hib					
Polio			Polio	Polio	Polio	Polio			Polio		
Measles, Mumps, Rubella						MMR	MMR		MMR	MMR	
Varicella						Var	Var			Var	

Quoted here without original notes from ACIP, AAP and AAFP .Approved by the Advisory Committee on Immunization Practices (ACIP), the American Academy of Pediatrics (AAP), and the American Academy of Family Physicians (AAFP).

TABLE 5

**Reported Cases of Vaccine-Preventable Diseases
January – November 1993-1994, U.S.**

Disease	Number of cases among children aged 5 and under for January - November	
	1993	1994
Congenital rubella syndrome	4	5
Diphtheria	0	1
*Hemophilus influenzae**	379	266
Hepatitis B**	120	106
Measles	114	211
Mumps	245	198
Pertussis	3,398	1,708
Poliomyelitis, paralytic	1	1
Rubella	31	21
Tetanus	0	0

* Invasive *Hemophilus influenzae* serotype is not routinely reported to the National Notifiable Diseases Surveillance System
** Because most hepatitis B virus infections among infants and children <5 years are asymptomatic (although likely to become chronic), acute disease surveillance does not reflect the incidence of this problem in this age group or the effectiveness of hepatitis B vaccination in infants.

SOURCE: From data released by Centers for Disease Control 1995.

TABLE 6

Law Enforcement, Courts, and Prisons
Child Abuse and Neglect Cases Reported and Investigated
1993-1994

Based on reports alleging child abuse and neglect that were referred for investigation by the respective child protective services agency in each State in the USA. The reporting period may be either calendar or fiscal year. The majority of States were unable to provide unduplicated counts. Only nine jurisdictions [Alaska, Hawaii, Michigan, Montana, Ohio, Oregon, South Carolina, Vermont, and Washington] provided unduplicated counts of children subject of report. Excludes the Armed Forces.

	1993 Reports				1994 Reports		
Population under 18 years old	Number of reports	Number of children subject of report	Investigation disposition, number of children substantiated	Population under 18 years old	Number of reports	Number of children subject of report	Investigation disposition, number of children substantiated
67,135,000	1,938,164	2,893,410	1,009,289	68,024,000	1,978,519	2,935,470	1,011,628

Reports are on incident/family-based basis or based on number of reported incidents regardless of the number of children involved in the incidents. Type of investigation disposition determines that there is sufficient evidence under State law to conclude that maltreatment occurred or that the child is at risk of maltreatment.

SOURCE: U.S. Department of Health and Human Services, National Center on Child Abuse and Neglect, National Child Abuse and Neglect Data System, Child Maltreatment – 1994.

TABLE 7

Juvenile Courts – Child Abuse and Neglect
Child Abuse and Neglect Cases Substantiated and Indicated – Victim Characterizations
1990-1994

Types of Substantiated Maltreatment	1990		1992		1993		1994	
	Number	Percent	Number	Percent	Number	Percent	Number	Percent
Victims, total*	761,153	(X)	1,054,456	(X)	1,067,231	100.0	1,197,133	100.0
Neglect	343,312	45.1	455,319	43.2	475,153	44.5	535,510	44.7
Physical Abuse	188,960	24.8	213,726	20.3	233,487	21.9	258,320	21.6
Sexual Abuse	120,732	15.9	130,739	12.4	139,817	13.1	139,980	11.7
Emotional Maltreatment	45,315	6.1	49,527	4.7	48,288	4.5	47,610	4.0
Medical Neglect	(NA)	(NA)	25,503	2.4	23,009	2.2	25,018	2.1
Other and Unknown	61,834	8.1	179,642	17.0	147,477	13.8	190,695	15.9

* More than one type of maltreatment may be substantiated per child. (X) = Not applicable. (NA) = Not Available

SOURCE: U.S. Department of Health and Human Services, National Center on Child Abuse and Neglect, National Child Abuse and Neglect Data System, Child Maltreatment – 1994.

TABLE 8

Juvenile Courts — Child Abuse and Neglect
Delinquency Cases Disposed by Juvenile Courts, by Reason for Referral: 1983-1993

In Thousands. A delinquency offense is an act committed by a juvenile for which an adult could be prosecuted in a criminal court. Disposition of a case involves taking a definite action such as transferring the case to criminal court, dismissing the case, placing the youth in a facility for delinquents, or such actions as fines, restitution, and community service.

REASON FOR REFERRAL	1983	1984	1985	1986	1987	1988	1989	1990	1991	1992	1993
All delinquency offences	1,030	1,034	1,112	1,150	1,156	1,170	1,212	1,299	1,407	1,460	1,490
Case rate*	38.3	38.7	42.2	43.9	44.5	45.7	47.8	51.0	53.9	54.7	54.6
VIOLENT OFFENSES	**55**	**61**	**67**	**73**	**67**	**71**	**78**	**95**	**109**	**118**	**122**
Criminal homicide	1	1	1	2	1	2	2	3	3	3	3
Forcible rape	3	3	4	5	4	4	4	4	5	5	6
Robbery	2	22	26	26	22	22	23	28	33	34	36
Aggravated Assault	27	35	36	40	39	43	49	60	69	77	78
PROPERTY OFFENSES	**451**	**442**	**489**	**496**	**498**	**501**	**525**	**546**	**601**	**595**	**573**
Burglary	145	129	139	140	131	129	131	143	155	156	150
Larceny	270	276	307	308	314	311	319	326	366	360	354
Motor vehicle theft	31	31	36	42	47	55	68	71	79	71	61
Arson	5	6	7	6	6	7	7	7	8	8	8
DELINQUENCY OFFENSES	**524**	**530**	**555**	**583**	**590**	**599**	**610**	**657**	**696**	**746**	**795**
Simple assault	81	73	92	95	100	104	110	125	137	152	166
Vandalism	64	69	84	84	83	81	83	97	111	117	117
Drug law violations	57	65	76	73	73	82	78	71	66	72	89
Obstruction of justice	55	63	68	76	79	79	82	86	82	86	96
Other**	268	260	235	255	256	253	256	278	301	320	327

*Number of cases disposed per 1,000 youth (ages 10 to 17) at risk. **Includes such offenses as stolen property offenses, trespassing, weapons offenses, other sex offenses, liquor law violations, disorderly conduct, and miscellaneous offenses.

SOURCE: National Center for Juvenile Justice, Pittsburgh, PA, Juvenile Court Statistics, annual.

FIGURE 1

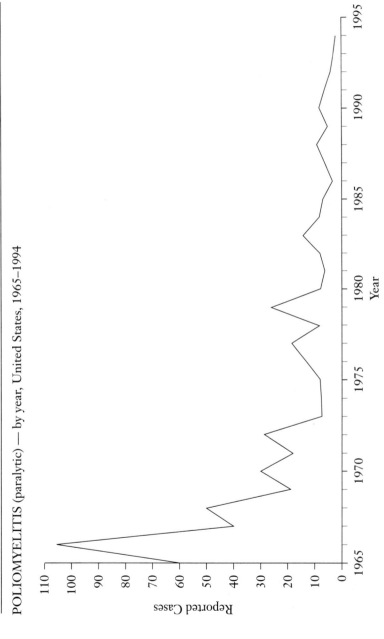

POLIOMYELITIS (paralytic) — by year, United States, 1965–1994

NOTE: Inactivated vaccine licensed 1955. Oral vaccine licensed 1961. Since 1980, all confirmed cases of indigenously acquired paralytic poliomyelitis in the United Staes have been vaccine associated.

SOURCE: U.S. Centers for Disease Control, CDC, Atlanta, Georgia

FIGURE 2

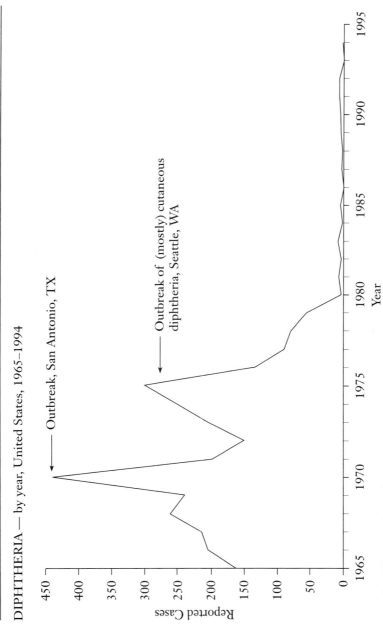

DIPHTHERIA — by year, United States, 1965–1994

Outbreak, San Antonio, TX

Outbreak of (mostly) cutaneous diphtheria, Seattle, WA

Reported Cases

Year

NOTE: DTP vaccine licensed 1949.

On ongoing epidemic of diphtheria is occuring in 14 of the 15 of the countries of the former Soviet Union. Two cases were reported among U.S. citizens residing in the former Soviet Union. No importation into the United States related to these outbreaks were reported in 1994.

SOURCE: U.S. Centers for Disease Control, CDC, Atlanta, Georgia

FIGURE 3

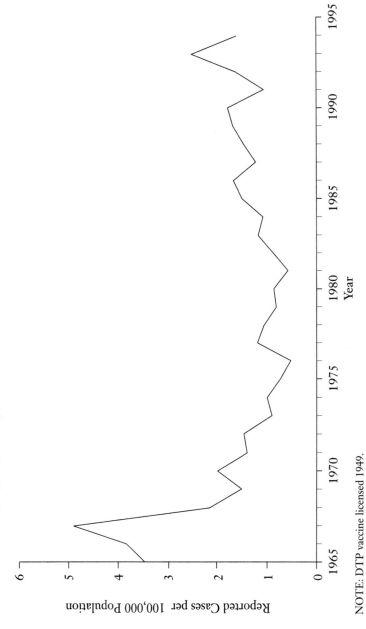

PERTUSSIS (whooping cough) — by year, United States, 1965–1994

Reported Cases per 100,000 Population

Year

NOTE: DTP vaccine licensed 1949.

The number of reported pertussis cases declined 30% from 1993–1994 — a pattern consistent with the previously observed 3- to 4-year periodicity in pertussis incidence.

SOURCE: U.S. Centers for Disease Control, CDC, Atlanta, Georgia

 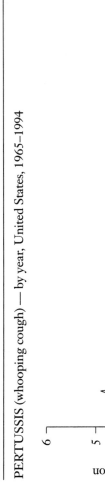

FIGURE 4

TETANUS — by year, United States, 1965–1994

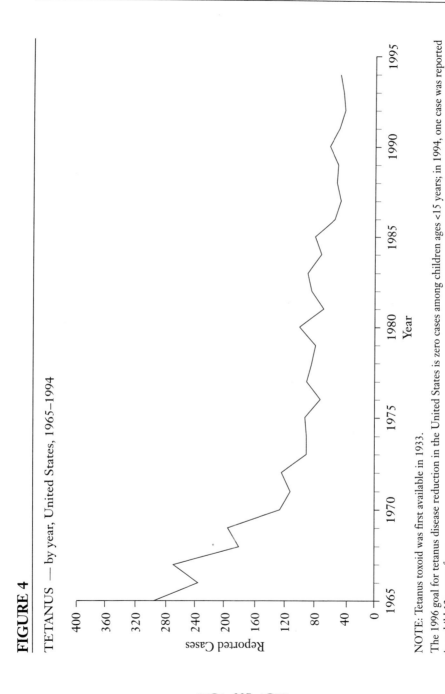

NOTE: Tetanus toxoid was first available in 1933.

The 1996 goal for tetanus disease reduction in the United States is zero cases among children ages <15 years; in 1994, one case was reported in a child 12 years of age.

SOURCE: U.S. Centers for Disease Control, CDC, Atlanta, Georgia

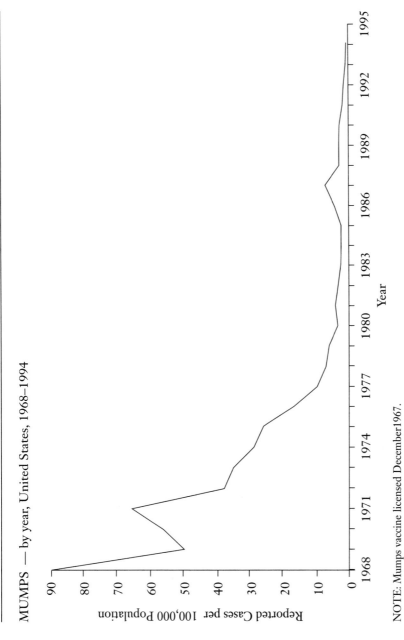

FIGURE 5

MUMPS — by year, United States, 1968–1994

NOTE: Mumps vaccine licensed December1967.

In 1994, 1,537 mumps cases were reported — the lowest number ever reported in the United States.

SOURCE: U.S. Centers for Disease Control, CDC, Atlanta, Georgia

FIGURE 6

MEASLES (rubeola) — by year, United States, 1950–1990

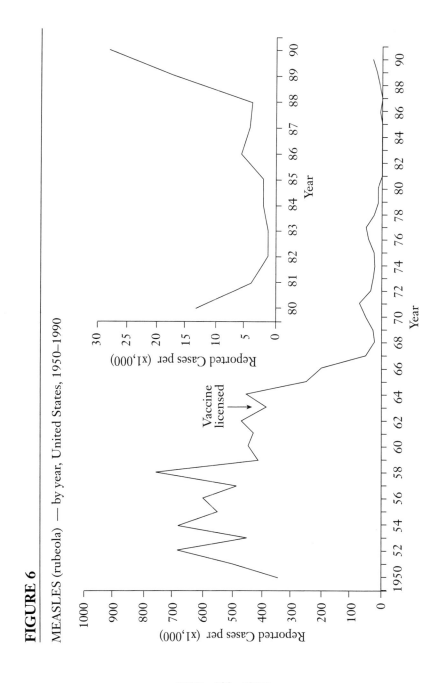

FIGURE 7

RUBELLA (German measles) — by year, United States, 1966–1994

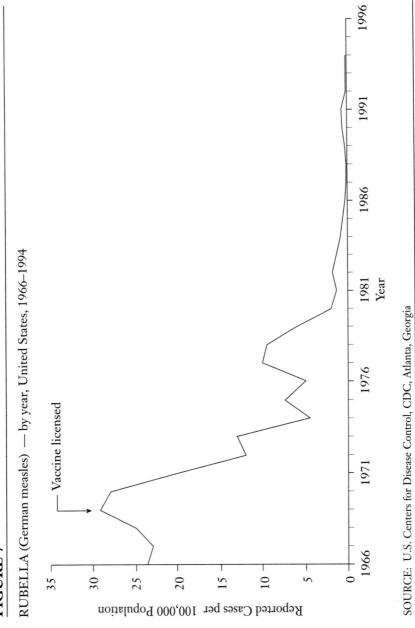

Vaccine licensed

Year

Reported Cases per 100,000 Population

SOURCE: U.S. Centers for Disease Control, CDC, Atlanta, Georgia